SO-BYE-046

Cardiovascular Nursing

nursing outline series

Rose Marie Greco, R.N., B.S.N., M.S.N.

Nursing Instructor
St. Louis Community College at Merramec
St. Louis, Missouri

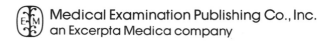

Medical Examination Publishing Co., Inc.
an Excerpta Medica company

Greco, Rose Marie.
    Cardiovascular nursing.

    (Nursing outline series)
    Bibliography: p.
    Includes index.
    1. Cardiovascular disease nursing. I. Title.
II. Series. [DNLM: 1. Cardiovascular diseases--
Nursing. WY 152.5 G791c]
RC674.G74   610.73'691   81-22375
ISBN 0-87488-403-9   AACR2

With much love to my parents

Catherine and William Urban

Contents

About the Author

Mrs. Greco received her diploma in Nursing from St. Luke's-Memorial Hospital School of Nursing, New Hartford, New York, a Bachelor of Science degree in Nursing at Avila College, Kansas City, Missouri, and a Master of Science degree in Nursing at the University of Missouri-Kansas City. Professional positions held include the following:

Presently Nursing Instructor, St. Louis Community College at Merramec, St. Louis, Missouri

Previous positions held:

Nurse Practitioner, Adult Medicine, Family Care Center of Carondolet, St. Louis, Missouri

Coordinator and Instructor, Medical-Surgical Nursing, Avila College, Kansas City, Missouri

Nurse Docent, Graduate Nursing Program, University of Missouri, Kansas City, Missouri

Inservice Instructor, Saint Joseph Hospital, Kansas City, Missouri

Staff Nurse, Female Admissions Unit, Marcy State Hospital, Marcy, New York

Staff and Charge Nurse, St. Luke's Memorial Hospital Center (Medical-Surgical Units, Pediatrics, Emergency Room, Intensive Care Unit), New Hartford, New York

Preface

Cardiovascular nursing is unique in its challenges and rewards. This book is designed to facilitate the effectiveness of administering nursing care to the adult client experiencing a cardiovascular alteration. This book will assist the nurse, nursing student, and other health care professionals in the delivery of safe, effective client care. Biologic and psychologic aspects of client care are considered. The text offers a concise, yet comprehensive review of current basic concepts of cardiovascular nursing. The nonsurgical approaches to cardiovascular nursing care of adult clients are stressed throughout the text. Although several traditional surgical interventions are briefly mentioned, readers interested in this aspect should refer to a text on cardiovascular surgery for a detailed description of the numerous, sophisticated techniques being utilized today.

Risk factors, warning signals, cardinal symptoms/signs, structure and function of the cardiovascular system, specialized diagnostic techniques, physical assessment, human sexuality, specific cardiovascular alterations, and the process of teaching and learning are included in this text. Learning objectives and review questions are grouped together for Parts I, II, and IV. Each chapter in Part III, which deals with specific alterations of the cardiovascular system, is preceded by specific learning objectives and the chapter is followed by review questions. References are included throughout the text to assist readers to further broaden their knowledge of specific topics and alterations of the cardiovascular system.

The appendix contains reference tables for the most commonly used cardiovascular drugs.

Acknowledgments

Many thanks to my husband, Frank, for his patience, understanding, and encouragement to continue and complete this work. Thanks and love to my children Anthony, Andrea, and Glorianne for their support and help at home during the research and writing process.

A special thank you to a longtime friend and advocate, Ardow Ameduri, M.D., who donated his time and effort to the task of proofreading the text. I would also like to acknowledge the assistance of Robert F. Schaefer, Registered Pharmacist, who took the time to review the drug section of the text.

Thanks to Richard Sanderson, M.D., W.B. Saunders Company, the American Heart Association, the Americal Journal of Nursing, Medical Examination Publishing Company, and Merck Sharp & Dohme Research Laboratories for providing me with invaluable reference materials.

notice

The author and the publisher of this book have made every effort to ensure that all therapeutic modalities that are recommended are in accordance with accepted standards at the time of publication.

The drugs specified within this book may not have specific approval by the Food and Drug Administration in regard to the indications and dosages that are recommended by the author. The manufacturer's package insert is the best source of current prescribing information.

PART I

INTRODUCTION

LEARNING OBJECTIVES

Study of Part I will enable the reader to:

1. Rank cardiovascular disease as a major cause of death in the United States

2. Identify cardiovascular risk factors that cannot be modified or eliminated

3. Describe risk factors that can be modified or eliminated

4. Recognize the warning signals of myocardial infarction

5. Discuss the "cardinal signs and symptoms" of cardiovascular disease

6. Demonstrate an ability to perform an accurate assessment of the client's pain

7. Summarize factors that place an additional strain on the heart; these factors may precipitate an attack of paroxysmal nocturnal dyspnea

8. Review the major causes of edema in clients experiencing a cardiovascular disease

9. State several noncardiac causes of edema

10. Assess the client for the "early signs" of edema

1

CHAPTER 1

MORTALITY, PREVALENCE, ECONOMIC COST, AND RISK FACTORS

MORTALITY

Cardiovascular disease continues to be the major cause of death in the United States today. In 1976, cardiovascular disease was responsible for 52% of all deaths (997, 766 deaths).[2] The American Heart Association estimated that 51% of all deaths, or approximately 980, 900 deaths in 1979, would be due to some form of cardiovascular disease. Approximately 25, 000 babies are born with heart defects annually. Although postnatal mortality from congenital heart defects has been reduced during the past several years, it is estimated that there were 6500 postnatal deaths from heart defects in 1979. [3] During 1979, heart attacks were responsible for approximately 549, 800 deaths. [3] Heart attack is still considered to be the nation's "Number One Killer. "[1] It is estimated that 4, 330, 000 people living today have a history of heart attack and/or angina pectoris. [3] Approximately 1. 5 million Americans are expected to have a heart attack (myocardial infarction) this year and about 550, 000 of these will die. [3] In 1979, stroke was responsible for about 169, 400 deaths. In the same year rheumatic heart disease and rheumatic fever resulted in approximately 7, 500 deaths. [3] However, mortality has decreased since the advent of antibiotics. It is thought that atherosclerosis contributed to many cases of heart attack and stroke in 1979.

PREVALENCE

The American Heart Association (AHA) reports that 41, 290, 000 Americans have some form of heart and blood vessel disease. [3] One in four adults is afflicted with hypertension, i. e. , approximately 35, 520, 000 Americans, many of whom are unaware of the condition. Of those who do know they have hypertension, many are not being adequately controlled. It is thought that approximately 4, 400, 000 people have coronary artery disease and 1, 920, 000 have rheumatic heart disease. Of those who have

3

rheumatic heart disease, approximately 100,000 are children; 1,820,000 are adults.[3] Stroke afflicts approximately 1,780,000.[3]

ECONOMIC COST

The American Heart Association estimates that cardiovascular disease will cost the nation approximately $50.7 billion in 1982.[3] This cost is $4.5 billion more than the estimate for 1981. Since 1949, it is estimated that more than $390 million have gone into research.[3] Hidden costs such as loss of job skills, job turnover, rehabilitation, etc. are difficult to establish.

RISK FACTORS

Some risk factors can be modified; others cannot. Risk factors that cannot be changed include heredity, sex, race, and age.[1]

There is no specific evidence that heredity increases the incidence of heart attack, stroke, or atherosclerosis; however, it is thought that a "tendency" toward these problems can be inherited. The death rate from heart attacks appears to be higher in males, but increases in females who are postmenopausal.

Black Americans are more likely to have hypertension than white. Since hypertension contributes to heart attack and stroke, and since blacks are afflicted with these conditions at earlier ages, many have detrimental effects from hypertension. Although it is thought that the rate of heart attacks increases as one gets older, many heart-attack deaths (one in four) occur in people under the age of 65 years. Stroke, once generally thought to afflict older persons, is now occurring in younger people (one in six deaths is under the age of 65 years).

Risk factors that can be modified or eliminated include such factors as smoking, hypertension, obesity, diabetes mellitus, hyperlipidemia, stress, and lack of exercise.[4]

The person who smokes more than 20 cigarettes per day has nearly twice the risk of heart attack. Since hypertension contributes to heart attacks and stroke, it is important to gain prompt "control" of the condition. A man with a systolic blood pressure of over 150 mm Hg has more than twice the risk of heart attack than a person with normal blood pressure. Obesity increases cardiac workload. Therefore, weight reduction should decrease cardiac work. There is a high incidence of coronary artery disease in persons who have diabetes mellitus. Diet regimens, weight control, and exercise programs help in controlling this condition. Hyperlipidemia (hypercholesterolemia and hypertriglyceridemia) is thought to predispose one to coronary artery disease. Dietary alterations can assist in returning these substances to normal ranges. Drugs also are available if dietary alterations alone are not effective. Prolonged stress may precipitate angina pectoris. The client must identify situations which are stress-producing and determine how these situations can be avoided or eliminated. It appears that men who lead sedentary lives are at greater risk of having heart attacks. Exercise programs should be initiated only after consultation with a physician.[1]

CHAPTER 2

WARNING SIGNALS, CARDINAL SYMPTOMS/SIGNS

WARNING SIGNALS

The American Heart Association defines the "signals" of heart attack as follows: an uncomfortable feeling of pressure, fullness, squeezing or pain in the center of the chest lasting two minutes or more; discomfort or pain radiating to the shoulders, neck, or arm; an uncomfortable feeling which may progress to severe pain and may be accompanied by dizziness, fainting, sweating, nausea, and dyspnea.[1]

CARDINAL SYMPTOMS/SIGNS OF CARDIOVASCULAR DISEASE/ ALTERATIONS

The six cardinal symptoms commonly identified in cardiovascular alterations include:

Chest Pain

Chest pain, one of the most common complaints, occurs in cardiovascular alterations such as: angina pectoris, myocardial infarction, pericardial effusion or tamponade, aortic dissection or aneurysm, and pulmonary embolism or infarction. Noncardiac disorders may also elicit chest pain and may make the diagnosis of heart disease more difficult. The noncardiac disorders include:

Arthritis of the lower or upper thoracic spine	Costochondritis
Cardiac neurosis	Periarthritis of the left shoulder
Sliding hiatus hernia	Spontaneous pneumothorax
Acute or chronic cholecystitis	Pleurisy
Acute pancreatitis	Spinal cord disease
Cardiospasm	Mediastinal tumor

6

Peptic ulcer

Esophageal pain

Neoplastic invasion of the ribs
    or vertebrae

Mediastinal emphysema[8]

A careful assessment of the client's pain should be carried
out. The nurse should ask the client to:

1. Describe the "quality" of the chest pain (sharp, dull, crushing, squeezing, etc.)

2. Identify the "location" of the chest pain

3. Estimate the "duration" of the pain

4. Determine points to which there is pain "radiation"

5. Describe "factors that precipitate, aggravate, or relieve the pain".[9] (A detailed symptom analysis can found on page 47.)

These data are utilized in the physician's final analysis of signs and symptoms to determine if the alteration is primarily of cardiac or noncardiac origin.

Dyspnea

Dyspnea is defined as "labored or difficult breathing"; this symptom is often described as "shortness of breath, " and is common to many diseases or alterations.[10] The symptom may be cardiac in origin, such as in left ventricular failure. Noncardiac causes of dyspnea include: poor physical condition, obesity, debility, advanced age, chronic lung disease, anemia, obstruction of the nasal passages, anxiety states, and cardiac neuroses.[8] There are several types of dyspnea or abnormal breathing patterns such as: exertional dyspnea, orthopnea, paroxysmal nocturnal dyspnea, cardiac asthma, and Cheyne-Stokes respirations.[9]

Exertional dyspnea is the most common type of cardiac dyspnea. The symptom occurs when the client exercises moderately and it is relieved when the client rests.

Orthopnea occurs when the client is lying flat in bed. The

symptom is relieved when the client sits upright. Orthopnea is considered to be more serious than exertional dyspnea, since it is indicative of advanced heart disease.[9]

Paroxysmal nocturnal dyspnea is another type of difficult breathing, which occurs periodically and suddenly at night. The client is awakened from sleep and has severe difficulty in breathing. Change of position, such as sitting or standing, helps to relieve the client. This type of dyspnea is most common in those cardiovascular conditions that overwork the left ventricle (hypertension, aortic stenosis, or aortic insufficiency).[9] Coughing, nightmares, abdominal distention, full bladder, heavy evening meal, or frightening noises are all factors which place an additional strain on the heart and may precipitate an attack of paroxysmal nocturnal dyspnea.[9] There may be several attacks during one night. Clients with cardiac asthma suffer from dyspnea and wheezing, which is related to pulmonary congestion and heart disease.[9] This symptom frequently occurs at night when the client is lying flat in bed.

Cheyne-Stokes respiration is a type of periodic breathing caused by diseases affecting the respiratory center, usually heart failure or brain damage.[10] The client's breathing is characterized by rhythmic waxing and waning of the depth of respiration; respirations may be deep, then become shallow and may cease completely for a short period. The pattern is repeated over and over.

Fatigue

Fatigue is considered to be an early symptom of heart disease. However, it is a common complaint which may arise from noncardiac causes. Fatigue may be the chief complaint in congenital heart disease, cor pulmonale, or mitral stenosis complicated by pulmonary hypertension.[8] The fatigue is improved by rest.

Psychologic disorders such as depression, cardiac neuroses, and chronic anxiety may cause fatigue which is unrelieved by rest. Other noncardiac causes of fatigue include infections, anemia, endocrine and metabolic disorders, chronic poisoning, chronic use of depressant or sedative drugs, malignancy, connective tissue diseases, and any other debilitating illness.[8]

Palpitation

Palpitation is a common symptom in clients who have organic heart disease. However, it is also commonly reported by clients whose cardiac symptoms have a neurotic basis.[9] The client usually states that he can feel his heart beating rapidly, forcefully, or irregularly, or that the heart is skipping or fluttering. Major causes of palpitations include: (1) nonfatal arrhythmias, (2) noncardiac organic problems such as anemia, hyperthyroidism, or infection, (3) nonpathologic factors such as excitement, exercise, alcohol, tobacco, excessive intake of coffee or tea, and (4) nervous and emotional disorders.[9]

Syncope

Syncope implies a temporary loss of consciousness which may or may not be preceded by dizziness.[11] It is the result of a sudden decrease in blood flow to the brain.[9] Cardiovascular causes of syncope include heart block; cardiac arrhythmias; severe aortic stenosis, on exertion; primary pulmonary hypertension, on exertion; idiopathic hypertrophic subaortic stenosis, after exertion; mitral valve obstruction; and prosthetic mitral or aortic valves that become occluded due to malfunction or formation of a thrombus.[6] Orthostatic hypotension and cerebral vascular disease (less common) may also cause syncope. Miscellaneous causes of syncope include: carotid sinus syndrome, glossopharyngeal neuralgia, micturation syncope, cough syncope, hysterical fainting, hypoglycemic episodes, and hyperventilation.[6]

Edema

Edema is indicative of a volume increase of the interstitial fluid, i.e., the extravascular portion of the extracellular compartment.[6] Edema of cardiac origin and heart failure appears first in the ankles and lower legs of ambulatory clients and over the sacrum, flanks, buttocks, and posterior thighs of bedridden clients.[8] Major causes of edema in clients with heart disease are:

1. Obstruction of blood into or from the heart

2. Fluid overload resulting in circulatory overload

3. Abnormal retention of water and electrolytes by the kidneys

4. Elevated renal, arterial, and venous pressure

5. Increased permeability of capillaries

6. A decrease in colloid osmotic pressure

7. Abnormalities in the formation and flow of lymph[9]

Noncardiac causes of edema include: obesity, incompetent leg veins, garters, rolled stockings, tight girdles, prolonged sitting/standing, premenstrual fluid retention, nephrosis, cirrhosis, congenital or acquired lymphedema, hypoprotein-emia, severe malnutrition or anemia, and obstruction of the inferior vena cava.[8]

The nurse should continually assess her cardiac client for early signs of edema noting any sudden weight gain; puffiness of the hands and ankles; or swelling over the sacrum, buttocks, or posterior thighs.[9]

Other signs and symptoms commonly seen in cardiovascular alterations include: intermittent claudication, cyanosis (late sign of oxygen deficiency), murmurs, distended neck veins, cough, and headache.[8, 9, 11]

REVIEW QUESTIONS TO PART I

1. How does cardiovascular disease rank as a major cause of death in the United States today?

2. Name four cardiovascular risk factors that <u>cannot</u> be changed.

3. Is the death rate from heart attacks (MI) greater in males or in females?

4. Are black or white Americans more likely to have hypertension?

5. Are heart attacks and strokes considered to be diseases or alterations of the elderly?

6. List seven cardiovascular risk factors which can be modified or eliminated.

7. What are the "signals" of heart attack published by the American Heart Association?

8. List the six cardinal symptoms of cardiovascular disease.

9. Which five items should be included in assessing the client's pain?

10. Define the following terms:

    Dyspnea   Paroxysmal nocturnal dyspnea

    Exertional dyspnea   Cheyne-Stokes respirations

    Orthopnea

11. Name six factors which may precipitate an attack of paroxysmal nocturnal dyspnea.

12. What are the major causes of edema in clients with heart disease?

13. List at least ten noncardiac causes of edema.

14. What "early signs of edema" would the nurse be looking for when assessing her client?

REFERENCES TO PART I

1. American Heart Association: Heart Facts 1978. American Heart Association Communications Division, 1977.

2. American Heart Association: 1979 Heart Facts Reference Sheet. American Heart Association Communications Division, 1978.

3. American Heart Association: Heart Facts 1982. American Heart Association Communications Division, 1981.

4. Boedeker, E. and Dauber, J.: Manual of Medical Therapeutics. 21st Ed., Boston: Little, Brown and Co., 1974, pp. 88-89.

5. Campbell, C. : Nursing Diagnosis and Intervention in Nursing Practice. New York: John Wiley and Sons, 1978, p. 22.

6. Friedman, H. H. (Ed.): Problem-Oriented Medical Diagnosis. Boston: Little, Brown and Co., 1975, pp. 384-387.

7. Gillies, D. A. and Alyn, I.: Patient Assessment and Management by the Nurse Practitioner. Philadelphia: W.B. Saunders Co., 1976, p. 30.

8. Krupp, M. A. and Chatton, M. J.: Current Medical Diagnosis and Treatment. Los Altos, Calif.: Lange Medical Publications, 1976, pp. 152-154.

9. Luckmann, J. and Sorensen, K.: Medical-Surgical Nursing, A Psychophysiologic Approach. Philadelphia: W.B. Saunders Co., 1974, pp. 612-616, 1980, pp. 777-780.

10. Miller, B. and Keane, C.: Encyclopedia and Dictionary of Medicine, Nursing and Allied Health. 2nd Ed., Philadelphia: W.B. Saunders Co., 1978, pp. 316, 200.

11. Silverman, M. E.: Examination of the Heart. Part I: The Clinical History. American Heart Association, Inc., 1975.

PART II

GENERAL NURSING CONSIDERATIONS

LEARNING OBJECTIVES

Study of Part II will enable the reader to:

1. Review the structure and function of the cardiovascular system

2. Discuss the specialized techniques used to establish a diagnosis of cardiovascular disease (noninvasive versus invasive techniques)

3. Prepare the client for various diagnostic procedures

4. Explain the techniques of inspection, palpation, percussion, and auscultation in relation to physical examination of the heart

5. Demonstrate the ability to perform a physical assessment of the client's cardiovascular system (historical data collection and physical examination)

6. State the screening questions that should be included in a historical review of the cardiovascular system for any client

7. Describe some of the practical approaches that can be used in performing a sexual assessment of a client with cardiovascular problems

8. Arrange for counseling sessions to assist the cardiac client to minimize cardiac work during sexual intercourse

15

CHAPTER 3

STRUCTURE AND FUNCTION OF THE CARDIOVASCULAR SYSTEM

Nurses caring for clients experiencing cardiovascular alterations must possess a solid knowledge base to understand the structure and function of the cardiovascular system. This knowledge base should be drawn upon during the application of the nursing process, which includes the phases of assessment, planning, intervention, and evaluation. The primary concern of the nurse is to assist the client in his adaptive responses (biologic and psychologic) to the alteration/illness.

THE HEART

The heart is often referred to as a "double pump. "[7, 26] It is a four-chambered, hollow, muscular organ located in the mediastinum lying between the lungs. Two-thirds of its mass is to the left of the midline. [23] Its approximate weight in a 150 lb male is 300 g and it is about the size of a man's fist. The heart's shape is often described as that of an inverted cone with its apex pointed downward toward the left; its base is directed toward the right side of the body. [23, 26] The structures of the heart include:

The Pericardium

The pericardium is the fibroserous sac enclosing the heart and the roots of the great vessels. [29] It consists of two layers: (1) an external fibrous layer called the parietal pericardium and (2) an internal serous layer which adheres to the heart called the visceral pericardium. [23] The internal serous layer also becomes the outermost layer of the heart called the epicardium. [23] Five to twenty milliliters of pericardial fluid is normally found in the pericardial space located between the two layers of the pericardium. [26] This fluid lubricates the two membranes as their surfaces glide over each other with each heart beat. [23]

Heart Wall

The heart wall consists of three layers: (1) the epicardium or external layer, which is the same structure as the visceral pericardium mentioned earlier; (2) the myocardium or middle layer is composed of striated muscle fibers, which enable the heart to contract and allow blood to be squeezed out of the heart and into the arterial system; and (3) the endocardium or inner layer, which is composed of endothelial tissue which lines the heart cavities, covers the valves, and is continuous with the lining of the large blood vessels. [23, 26]

Heart Chambers

The heart has four chambers. There are two upper or receiving chambers called the atria. The right and left atria are separated by the interatrial septum. The atria receive blood from different parts of the body and pump blood into the ventricles. [23] The two lower or distributing chambers are called the ventricles. The right and left ventricles are separated by the interventricular septum. [23] The ventricles distribute or pump blood to the lungs and other parts of the body (See Figure 1).

The right atrium in the right superior portion of the heart is a thin-walled chamber, which receives blood from all body tissues except the lungs. [23] The three veins that drain into the right atrium are the: (1) superior vena cava, (2) inferior vena cava, and (3) coronary sinus. The right ventricle makes up the right inferior portion of the heart apex. [23]

The pulmonary artery leaves the right ventricle from its superior surface carrying blood to the lungs. [23] The left atrium comprises the left superior portion of the heart. [23] Although it is slightly smaller than the right atrium, it has a thicker wall. The left atrium receives oxygenated blood from the lungs through the four pulmonary veins. [23]

The left inferior portion of the apex of the heart is taken up by the left ventricle. The walls of the left ventricle are three times as thick as the walls of the right ventricle. The left ventricle pumps blood to all parts of the body, except the lungs, through the aorta. [23]

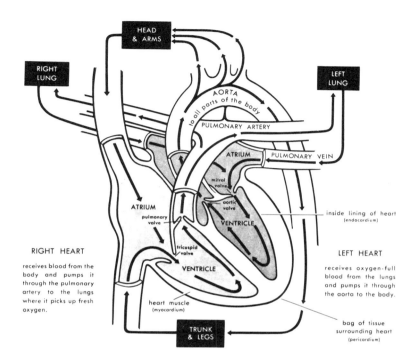

Figure 1. Your Heart and How It Works. (Reprinted with permission © American Heart Association.)

Heart Valves

Two types of valves are located in the heart: (1) the atrioventricular valves, called the tricuspid and the mitral valves, located between the atria and the ventricles, respectively, and (2) the semilunar valves, called the pulmonic and the aortic valves, located at the point at which the pulmonary artery and the aorta leave the ventricles. [23]

The tricuspid valve, on the right side of the heart, consists of three irregularly shaped cusps, whose ends project

into the ventricle and are attached by the chordae tendineae
to the papillary muscles within the inside of the ventricle. The
mitral valve guards the left atrioventricular opening and consists of two cusps. [23] The mitral valve is stronger and thicker
than the tricuspid valve and is attached in the same manner.
When the two atria contract, blood passes through the tricuspid
and mitral valves and fills the ventricles. When the ventricles
contract, these valves are closed by the union of the cusps.
This prevents blood from being forced backward from the ventricles to the atria. [23, 26]

The pulmonary semilunar valve, which is located between
the pulmonary artery and the right ventricle, prevents blood
from flowing back into the right ventricle from the pulmonary
artery. The aortic semilunar valve, which lies between the
aorta and the left ventricle, prevents blood from flowing back
into the left ventricle from the aorta. [23]

Heart sounds are caused by the closure of the heart valves.
Note the location of the valve areas in Figure 2. The first
heart sound (S1), described by the syllable "lubb, " occurs at
the beginning of ventricular systole and is caused by the closure of the tricuspid and mitral valves. [23] The second heart
sound (S2) is classically described by the syllable "dubb" and
is produced by the closure of the pulmonic and the aortic semilunar valves at the end of systole or beginning of diastole. [23]
Refer to Figure 3 for a graphic representation of heart sounds.

CORONARY BLOOD SUPPLY

The right and left coronary arteries which are the first
branches of the aorta supply blood to the whole myocardium. [23]
The right coronary artery branches to the sinus node in over
50% of hearts and to the right atrium and ventricle. The right
coronary artery turns posteriorly around the inferior margin
of the heart and sends branches to the atrioventricular (AV)
node, bundle of His, and the posterior division of the left bundle branch. [7] The posterior descending branch supplies nearly
half of the inferior surface of the left ventricle. [7] The left
coronary artery divides into the circumflex artery and the
anterior descending branch. The circumflex artery supplies
blood to the left atrium and left ventricle. The anterior descending branch supplies blood to the left and right ventricles. [23]

The left ventricle is drained by the largest system of coronary veins: the coronary sinus and its tributaries. [7] The right

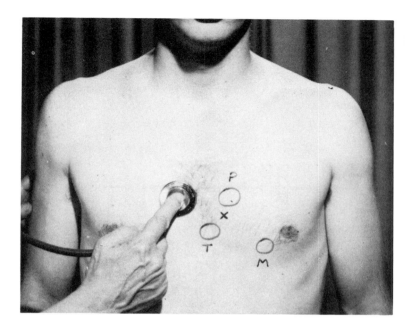

Figure 2. Cardiac auscultation. Circles mark the valve areas, according to the old poem, "Aortic right, Pulmonic left, Tricuspid's 'neath the sternum, Mitral's at the apex beat, And that is how we learn 'em." Erb's point is marked by an X. (Reprinted with permission from Sherman, J. and Fields, S.: Guide to Patient Evaluation. Garden City, NY: Medical Examination Publishing Co., Inc., 1978, p. 181.)

ventricle is drained by the anterior cardiac veins which empty into the right atrium.[7]

The smallest system of veins called the "thebesian veins" are found primarily in the right atrium and right ventricle. These veins drain directly into the cardiac chambers[7] (See Figure 4).

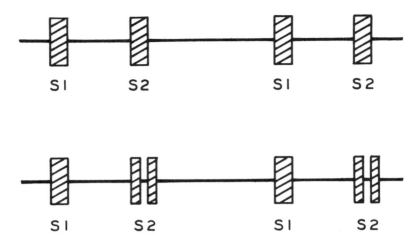

Figure 3. Graphic representation of heart sounds. The upper line is normal. The lower represents a split second sound. Note the closeness of the two components of the split sound. Systole is the interval between S1 and S2; diastole occurs between S2 and the next S1. (Reprinted with permission from Sherman, J. and Fields, S.: Guide to Patient Evaluation. Garden City, NY: Medical Examination Publishing Co., Inc., 1978, p. 185.)

CARDIAC MUSCLE

Certain properties of cardiac muscle are essential for the regulation of the heart rate and rhythm. These properties include:

Rhythmicity

The heart has the ability to beat without external stimuli and it possesses a rhythm in both formation and conduction of electrical impulses from atria to ventricles.[26, 29]

Irritability

Cardiac muscle cells have the ability to respond to stimuli. The irritable heart muscle responds to stimuli with the strongest possible contraction ("all-or-none law").[26]

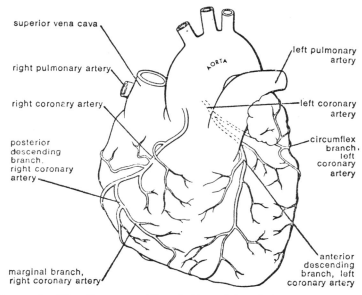

Figure 4. The Coronary Circulation. (Reprinted with permission © The American Heart Association.)

Refractoriness

This property helps to preserve heart rhythm because it prevents heart muscle from responding to a new stimulus while it is still in a state of contraction due to a previous stimulus. During the "absolute refractory period," the heart muscle does not respond to any stimulus.[26]

Conductivity

Heart muscle fibers have the ability to conduct or transmit electrical impulses.[26]

Contractility

Heart muscle fibers have the capacity to shorten in response to suitable stimuli.[26]

Automaticity

The heart has the ability to beat spontaneously and repetitively without external neurohormonal control.

Extensibility

Heart muscle has the ability to stretch as the heart is being filled with blood during diastole.[26] Starling's "Law of the Heart" states that, "The energy of contraction is proportional to the initial length of the cardiac fiber."[23] The greater the initial length of the muscle fibers, the more forceful will be the contraction. Overstretching of fibers, however, results in a weak contraction.[23]

NERVOUS CONTROL OF THE HEART

The two divisions of the autonomic nervous system control the heart: (1) the parasympathetic nervous system (the vagus) and (2) the sympathetic nervous system. The vagus nerve acts as a cardiac inhibitor[23] (i.e., the vagus causes a slowing of the rate of firing of the sinus node and a decrease in the rate of conduction through the AV node).[7] Stimulation of the sympathetic nerves can: (1) cause increased force of cardiac contraction, (2) enhance excitability of the heart, and (3) increase the rate of the sinus node.[7]

CONDUCTION SYSTEM

The cardiac conduction system is comprised of specialized cardiac muscle cells which have the ability to: (1) initiate the sequence of events in the cardiac cycle and (2) control the cycle's regularity.[23, 26] The conduction system is comprised of the following structures:

Sinoatrial Node

The sinoatrial (SA) node is located at the junction of the superior vena cava and the right atrium. This node is often referred to as the "pacemaker" of the heart because its regular rate of electrical discharge sets the rhythm of contraction for the entire heart.[23, 26] The firing rate of the sinoatrial node is between 60 to 100 beats per minute. Specialized tissue in the atria, ventricles, and AV node can assume the role of pacemaker, if they initiate impulses at a faster rate than the SA node.

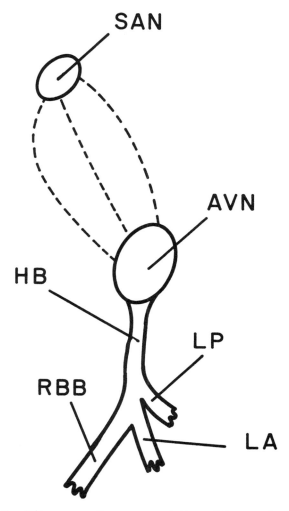

Figure 5. Diagrammatic representation of the conduction system. SAN = sinoatrial node, AVN = atrioventricular node, HB = His bundle, LA = anterior fascicles of the left bundle branch, LP = posterior fascicles of the left bundle branch, RBB = right bundle branch. Dashed lines indicate internodal tracts. (Reprinted with permission from Anthony, C. et al.: Pediatric Cardiology — Medical Outline Series. Garden City, NY: Medical Examination Publishing Co., Inc., 1979, p. 56).

Atrioventricular Node

The atrioventricular (AV) node is located in the right posterior portion of the interatrial septum.[23] The AV node receives electrical impulses from the SA node; the impulse is delayed briefly and is then transmitted to the bundle of His.[23,26]

Bundle of His-Purkinje System

This system is continuous with the AV node.[26] The bundle of His relays impulses from the AV node to the ventricle. The Purkinje fibers assist in the rapid spread of electrical impulses over all parts of the ventricles. Figure 5 is a diagrammatic representation of the conduction system.

BLOOD VESSELS

Blood vessels are classified as: (1) large or elastic arteries, (2) medium-sized or muscular arteries, (3) small arteries or arterioles, (4) capillaries, and (5) veins.[23]

The blood vessels are composed of three layers: a tunica adventitia (the outer coat); a tunica media (the middle coat); and a tunica intima (the innermost coat, also called Bichat's tunic).[29] The arteries are the thickest blood vessels, since muscular walls are necessary for contraction to transport blood from the heart to the capillaries. Capillary walls are one cell layer thick. This allows for the exchange of carbon dioxide and oxygen in the lungs and nutrients and wastes in the body.[23] Capillaries containing deoxygenated blood unite to form veins. The veins return the blood to the heart. Veins are characterized by valves, which prevent the backflow of blood.[23]

CHAPTER 4

SPECIALIZED TECHNIQUES UTILIZED TO ESTABLISH A DIAGNOSIS

ECHOCARDIOGRAPHY

Echocardiography is a type of noninvasive diagnostic technique, which is based upon the principle of ultrasound. Ultrasonic rays are reflected from the interspaces between the heart wall and the surrounding tissue or cardiac valves and blood, and travel back toward the transducer, which also acts as a receiver.[4, 32] The ultrasonic signals obtained from the cardiac structures are displayed on an oscilloscope and permanent records on film or paper strips can be made. Cardiac structures can be identified by assessing the appearance, position, motion pattern, and intensity of echo signals derived from them, as well as their relationship to other recognized structures.[32]

Echocardiography can be used as a diagnostic tool for clients with: mitral stenosis, idiopathic hypertrophic subaortic stenosis (IHSS), prolapsed mitral valve, torn chordae tendineae, vegetations due to bacterial endocarditis, aortic insufficiency, and pericardial effusion.[20] Echocardiography also can be used to evaluate the left ventricle in regard to chamber size and function.

The client should be advised that the procedure is painless. Clients may be permitted to eat and drink before testing and no sedation is necessary.

PHONOCARDIOGRAPHY

This noninvasive technique, which utilizes a transducer and a microphone, permits the recording of audible vibrations from the heart and great vessels. It may be considered as an extension of cardiac auscultation and is useful in documenting physical findings. A transducer is applied first to the apical region and then to the tricuspid, pulmonic, and aortic areas of

27

the heart. A permanent record of the occurrence, timing, and duration of the sounds of the cardiac cycle is obtained. [4] Low frequency sounds which may not be audible with the stethoscope can be recorded. No special client preparation is required. As with all procedures, the client should receive a detailed description of the procedure and its purposes.

EXERCISE TESTING

This diagnostic procedure is sometimes referred to as the stress test, exercise electrocardiography, or the treadmill test. This test allows evaluation of physical performance capacity in a controlled setting with electrocardiographic monitoring during the exercise test. [4] When the treadmill is used, the speed and inclination are increased at intervals to produce a graded work load. The test is terminated if serious ECG changes, shortness of breath, or pain occur.

ELECTROCARDIOGRAM

The electrocardiogram is another noninvasive diagnostic technique, which is considered to be an essential tool in the evaluation of cardiac status. It is a graphic record of the electric impulses generated by depolarization and repolarization of the myocardium. [26] The electrocardiogram (ECG) requires the placement of electrodes on the body to pick up electric current. The electric events of the cardiac cycle are visible on an ECG strip or on an oscilloscope. [4]

Leads

A standard ECG involves the recording of 12 leads. Each lead allows for the heart to be viewed from a different direction. There are three bipolar limb leads: leads I, II, and III.

Lead I records the difference in voltage between the right arm (the negative electrode) and the left arm (the positive electrode).

Lead II records the difference in voltage between the right arm (negative lead) and the left leg (positive lead).

Lead III records the difference in voltage between the left arm (negative lead) and the left leg (positive lead). [2]

The axis of the three bipolar limb leads forms a triangle with its tip at the lower part of the body and the heart as its center. This triangle is often referred to as the Einthoven triangle. There are three augmented unipolar limb leads: aV_R (right arm), aV_L (left arm), and aV_F (foot). These leads determine the electric potentials at single lead sites and are relatively uninfluenced by a reference to another electrode. "The unipolar lead compares the electrical potentials of the heart with zero. "[7]

There are six precordial or chest leads, which are also unipolar: V_1, V_2, V_3, V_4, V_5, V_6 (see Figure 6 for the precordial electrode positions).

WAVES OF EXCITATION

The waves of excitation seen on the ECG strip were arbitrarily designated the letters P, Q, R, S, T (illustrated in Figure 10). [7, 26]

P Wave

The P wave represents atrial depolarization; the duration of the wave is normally about 0.08 second. The P wave deflection is small (not more than 3 mm in height) because the atrial wall is relatively thin. A positive deflection is usually seen in leads I, II, and aV_F because the current is flowing toward the positive terminals. [7] Deflections of the P wave in aV_L and V_3 to V_6 may be positive, negative, or diphasic. The P wave in leads III, V_1, and V_2 may be upright, diphasic, flat, or inverted depending on the heart's position in the body and on the orientation of the atrial vector to the positive terminals; the P wave is normally inverted in aV_R. [7] (See Figure 7 for the generation of the normal P wave.)

PR Interval

The PR interval represents the time necessary for the impulse to spread from the atria to the ventricles. The average duration of the PR interval is 0.16 second; it should be no less than 0.12 second or more than 0.20 second. [8, 26]

QRS Complex

The QRS complex represents ventricular depolarization or the time it takes for the ventricles to depolarize. See Figures

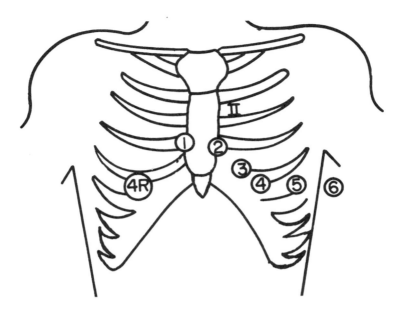

Figure 6. Precordial electrode positions. Leads V1 and V2
are recorded in the fourth intercostal space at the right and
left sternal borders respectively. V4 is in the left fifth intercostal space at the midclavicular line; V3 is located at the mid-
point of a line connecting V2 and V4. V5 and V6 are at the
same level as V4 in the anterior and midaxillary lines respectively. V4R is in the same position as V4 over the right
hemithorax. (Reprinted with permission from Anthony, C.,
et al.: Pediatric Cardiology — Medical Outline Series.
Garden City, NY: Medical Examination Publishing Co., Inc.,
1979, p. 55).

8 and 9 which demonstrate the sequence of ventricular depolarization in the generation of the QRS complex.

The QRS complex usually consists of three separate waves
created by the passage of the cardiac electrical impulse through
the ventricles. At times, the three waves may not be present,
but the complex is still referred to as the QRS complex.

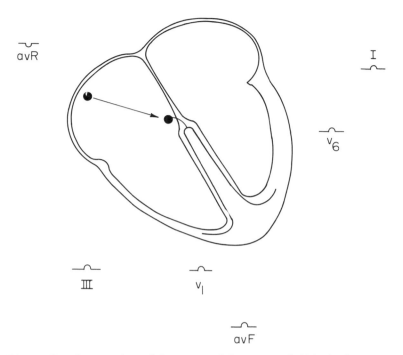

avR

I

v₆

III

vᵢ

avF

Figure 7. Generation of the normal P wave. Solid circles represent sinoatrial and atrioventricular nodes. Overall leftward, inferior, and anterior direction of spread of the atrial excitation wave results in P wave configuration as shown in selected leads. (Reprinted with permission from Anthony, C. et al.: Pediatric Cardiology — Medical Outline Series. Garden City, NY: Medical Examination Publishing Co., Inc., 1979, p. 57.)

The QRS complex occurs at the beginning of ventricular contraction.[29] Normally, the R wave is the most prominent of the three waves; the Q and S waves may be weak or absent. The voltage of the QRS complex may be increased as a result of hypertrophy of the cardiac muscle caused by excessive work load. A decrease in the voltage of the QRS complex may result in the pericardium, pleural effusion, and emphysema.[29] The normal duration of the QRS complex is usually given as 0.05 to 0.10 second.[8]

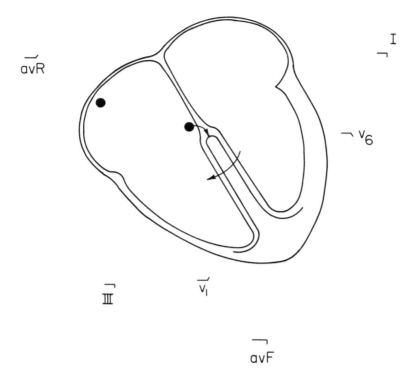

Figure 8. Early phase of ventricular depolarization. The interventricular septum is depolarized from left to right side
producing the deflections shown in the initial part of the QRS
complex. (Reprinted with permission from Anthony, C. et al. :
Pediatric Cardiology — Medical Outline Series. Garden City,
NY: Medical Examination Publishing Co., Inc., 1979, p. 58.)

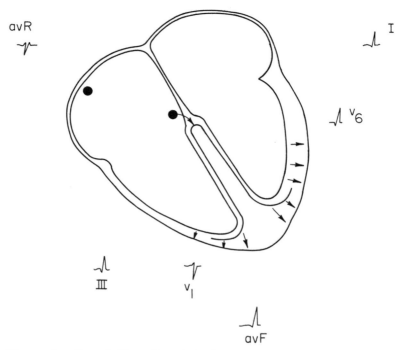

Figure 9.   Completion of ventricular depolarization.   As a result of greater myocardial mass of the left ventricle, the net forces are directed leftward, posteriorly, and inferiorly. (Reprinted with permission from Anthony, C. et al.: Pediatric Cardiology — Medical Outline Series. Garden City, NY: Medical Examination Publishing Co., Inc., 1979, p. 59.)

ST Segment

The ST segment signifies that ventricular depolarization is complete and repolarization is about to begin. Duration of the ST segment is approximately 0.12 second.[26]

QT Interval

The QT interval ventricular contraction occurs essentially between the Q wave and the end of the T wave; it is approximately 0.30 second.[18] The QT interval is primarily equal to the refractory period of the heart and therefore changes with heart rate.[7] Prolongation of the QT interval may be the result of myocardial ischemia, quinidine, and hypocalcemia.[7] The QT interval may be shortened with digitalis, propranolol, phenytoin, and hypercalcemia.[7] It is often felt that the QT interval is not as reliable a measurement as the other waves mentioned in this section.

T Wave

The T wave indicates repolarization of the ventricles. The duration of the T wave is approximately 0.16 second.[26] A stimulus during the T wave may precipitate a serious ventricular arrhythmia. This is especially likely if the stimulus occurs during the vulnerable period.

LABORATORY TESTS

The role of the nurse in today's society is continuously expanding. As the responsibilities increase, so must the nurse's knowledge base expand or increase so that nursing judgments are based upon sound rationale. This necessitates a knowledge

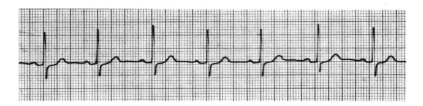

Figure 10. Normal sinus rhythm at a rate of 75 per minute. (Reprinted with permission from Sanderson, R.G.: The Cardiac Patient. Philadelphia: W.B. Saunders Co., 1972.)

of the purposes, functions, and significance of laboratory studies. This acquired knowledge base prepares the nurse to exercise judgment in the interpretation of laboratory studies in relation to other client data such as history, subjective data (symptoms), objective data (signs), electrocardiographic pattern, and adaptive responses to the alteration experienced.[22, 37]

SERUM ENZYME STUDIES

Enzymes are proteins found in all living cells which serve as accelerating agents or catalysts for chemical reactions.[22, 37] Different enzymes are found in different types of cells. Overactive, diseased, or injured cells increase the release of their enzymes into the serum. [22] The difference in composition and concentration of the various enzymes in different tissues permits the use of serum enzyme determinations to assist in the detection of specific cell damage (cardiac, liver, skeletal muscle, brain, etc.). It is important to remember that there is no one serum enzyme elevation that is diagnostic of any one disease. [22] Cardiac enzymes which occur in, and are released in, proportionately larger amounts from cardiac tissue include:

Creatine phosphokinase (CPK)

Hydroxybutyric dehydrogenase (HBD)

Serum glutamicoxaloacetic transaminase (SGOT)

Lactic dehydrogenase (LDH)

It is important to remember that enzymes are evaluated by a variety of laboratory methods and the determinations are reported in different quantitative units. Therefore, the "normal ranges" will vary according to the procedures used by a particular laboratory. The nurse should become acquainted with the range of normals for each enzyme at the specific facility where he/she is employed.

CPK

CPK rises and falls faster than the other cardiac enzymes (see Table 1). Because of the transient nature of the elevation, the CPK rise may be completely missed if the client delays hospitalization and seeking medical advice. CPK is found in brain tissue and skeletal and cardiac muscle. [22] Conditions causing a rise in CPK levels are myocardial infarction, acute cerebrovascular disease, muscular dystrophy, muscle trauma, peripheral arterial embolism, repeated intramuscular injections, and operative procedures.[22] CPK can be fractionated into three isoenzymes: (1) CPK-MM, a fast-acting isoenzyme found in skeletal muscle; (2) CPK-MB, an intermediate-acting isoenzyme found in the myocardium; and (3) CPK-BB, a slow-acting isoenzyme found in brain tissue. The source of CPK elevation can be very helpful in establishing a diagnosis.

LDH

"Total" LDH is probably the least specific for cardiac disease because of its abundance in kidney, heart, liver, muscle tissues, and red cells.[22] Table 1 shows time of onset and duration of elevation after myocardial infarction. Because the LDH does not return to normal for 7 to 11 days, it may be helpful in making a late diagnosis. Five isoenzymes (different molecular forms that catalyze the same chemical reaction) of LDH can be recognized electrophoretically.[33] These five isoenzymes range from fastest acting to slowest acting:

LDH_1 and LDH_2:   the faster isoenzymes, found in cardiac muscle, renal cortex, erythrocytes, and the cerebrum

LDH_3:   an intermediate-acting isoenzyme, found in the spleen, leukocytes, pancreas, and lung tissue

Table 1. Cardiac Enzyme Elevations Following Myocardial Infarction[22, 37]

Total	Onset of Elevation (hr)	Peak Elevation (hr)	Return to Normal (days)
LDH	12-24 after tissue damage	72 (3 x normal)	7-11
CPK	2-5	12-36 (5-12 x normal)	2-3
SGOT	6-12	18-36 (5 x normal, but may go up with extensive infarct)	4-6

LDH$_4$ and LDH$_5$: the slowest-acting isoenzymes, found
in liver, skeletal muscle, and spleen

The activity of LDH$_2$ in the serum is normally greater
than LDH$_1$. In an acute myocardial infarction (MI), LDH$_1$ is
liberated as a result of myocardial necrosis and, therefore,
the LDH$_1$ level becomes higher than LDH$_2$. This is called a
"flipped" pattern and occurs one to three days following myocardial infarction.[37] During the initial 48 hours after an acute
MI, the presence of CPK-MB isoenzyme in conjunction with a
flipped LDH pattern is considered diagnostic for myocardial
infarction.[37]

SGOT

Tissue distribution of SGOT is widespread and is found in
large amounts in red cells, liver, renal tissue, and cardiac
and skeletal muscle; lesser amounts are found in the brain,
pancreas, and lung tissue. SGOT is one of the least specific
enzymes, second to total LDH.[22] SGOT elevations are seen in
clients experiencing tachyarrhythmias (with or without MI),
liver damage from congestive heart failure, acute liver damage
after alcohol ingestion, shock, pericarditis, dissecting aortic
aneurysm, excessive vigorous exercise, trauma, cerebral
infarction, acute cholecystitis, pancreatitis, pulmonary infarction, and drugs such as narcotics and anticoagulants.[22]

If myocardial infarction has occurred, all the enzymes
should be elevated between 24 to 48 hours after symptoms have
occurred.[22] If serum enzyme levels have remained normal
for 36 to 48 hours after the occurrence of symptoms, one can
assume that MI has not occurred.

OTHER LABORATORY TESTS

Erythrocyte count and hemoglobin concentration are done
to evaluate the oxygen-carrying capacity of the blood. Normal
values:

Red blood cell count: Males   4.8 to 5.4 million/cm
                        Females 4.5 to 5.0 million/cm

Hemoglobin: Males   14 to 18 g/100 ml blood
                        Females 12 to 16 g/100 ml blood[4]

Leukocyte count is done to determine if an inflammatory process is present. The leukocyte count is elevated after an MI in response to the inflammatory process. The normal range for white blood cells is 5000 to 10, 000/cu mm. [4]

Electrolyte levels along with the hematocrit can be used to determine the fluid and electrolyte status of the client. The serum potassium is elevated when cellular damage occurs and potassium (K^+) is released from the cells. Levels of intracellular K^+ are decreased after MI. Potassium supplements may be required to prevent hypokalemia and arrhythmias. Low K^+ levels can cause digitalis toxicity in clients receiving digitalis-- serious arrhythmias can result. Sodium retention is associated with congestive heart failure and results in elevated levels of serum sodium. Clients receiving excessive dosages of diuretics and restricted sodium diets may have dangerously decreased sodium and K^+ levels. [4]

Erythrocyte sedimentation rate is done to determine the rate at which erythrocytes settle in a column of blood. Increased sedimentation rates are associated with inflammatory processes such as rheumatic fever, post-MI, and other non-cardiac conditions. [4]

Serum lipids and plasma lipoprotein patterns which show a total blood cholesterol level higher than 250 mg/100 ml of blood suggest that atherosclerosis is present. Phospholipids and triglycerides are also evaluated. Determination of lipoprotein patterns allows for classification of the type of hyper-lipoproteinemia present. [4]

Blood urea nitrogen (BUN) may be elevated due to inadequate cardiac function, which decreases the blood supply to the kidneys. [4]

Blood glucose is important because the incidence of coronary heart disease is higher in clients who have diabetes and elevated glucose levels, than in clients whose glucose levels are normal. [4]

Prothrombin time and clotting time are often done to obtain baseline data for normal clotting mechanisms in the event that anticoagulant therapy becomes necessary. Some clients with cardiovascular alterations already may be on anticoagulants at the time of admission. [4]

<u>Blood culture</u> is done to detect the presence of bacteria in the circulating blood. The test is indicated especially if bacterial endocarditis is suspected.[4]

<u>Antistreptolysin O titer</u> is used to determine whether a client with possible rheumatic heart disease has had a recent infection; it measures the presence and amount of antibodies against streptolysin O (the streptococcal enzyme), which destroys erythrocytes.

<u>Arterial blood gas</u> analyzes for the oxygen, carbon dioxide, and <u>pH levels</u> of arterial blood.[4]

<u>Urinalysis</u> is done because abnormal amounts of albumin may be present in congestive heart failure.[4]

CHEST X-RAY

Posteroanterior and lateral chest films are done to demonstrate heart size and status of the vascular bed in the lung fields.[4]

VENOUS PRESSURE MEASUREMENTS

Central Venous Pressure

The central venous pressure (CVP) refers to the pressure or force exerted by the blood in the right atrium or superior vena cava.[19, 22] The CVP measurement provides relative information regarding the following parameters: (1) pumping action of the heart, (2) blood volume, and (3) vascular tone.[19, 22] The CVP line consists of an intravenous catheter positioned in the superior vena cava or right atrium.[19] The catheter is attached to a closed system of IV tubing and a manometer calibrated in centimeters. The CVP measurement is done with the client in the supine position with the head of the bed flat unless contraindicated by the client's condition. If the head of the bed must be elevated, each measurement should be taken with the head of the bed at the <u>same</u> elevation. The catheter is inserted into the client's right <u>atrium</u> via the superior vena cava by the physician. The zero point of the manometer should be placed along the lateral chest wall at the level of the client's right atrium along the midaxillary line about 5 cm posterior to the sternum wall at the second intercostal space.[12] The external reference point for the right atrium, an "X, " should be marked with a marking pen, so that all persons caring for the client

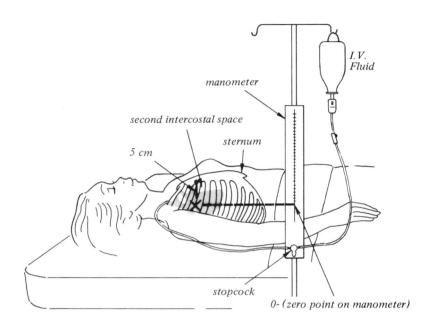

Figure 11. The external reference point for the right atrium, an "X," should be marked with a marking pen, so that all persons caring for the client may use the same reference point. The zero point of the manometer should be placed along the lateral chest wall at the level of the client's right atrium along the midaxillary line about 5 cm posterior to the sternal wall at the second intercostal space.

may use the same reference point (See Figure 11). The exact procedure for CVP measurement usually can be found on the box panel which contains the sterile IV tubing and the three-way stopcock, or in any of the hospital's nursing procedure books. The technique may vary slightly from facility to facility.

Clients on ventilators pose special problems since the ventilator's positive pressure will cause falsely elevated CVP readings. If the client can tolerate it, the physician may allow him to be taken off the ventilator for readings. If the client must remain on the ventilator, this should be recorded and all other readings should be taken in this manner.

Physicians disagree regarding the normal range for the CVP. Normal range may vary from -2 to 7 mm H_2O, 8 to 10 is borderline and 13 to 15 is considered abnormal. [16] Numerous other figures are stated in the literature for normal CVP readings. The nurse should remember that a single reading is not as significant as the trend of the CVP. [19] The CVP reading is lower than usual when the blood volume is reduced and the reading is elevated when the circulatory system is overloaded. [26] The CVP can be estimated by examining the cervical veins and the veins on the back of the client's hand. Sepsis can be a serious complication of CVP monitoring due to: (1) contaminated IV tubing, (2) bacterial invasion of the insertion site, and (3) break in aseptic technique in handling equipment and dressing changes. [19] The nurse making the changes should label all new dressings and tubing showing the date and time of change and the nurse's initials. [12]

Pulmonary Artery Pressure

The pulmonary artery pressure (PAP) reflects left ventricular function. The pulmonary artery (PA) and the mean pulmonary-capillary wedge (PCW) pressures can be obtained by inserting a flow-directed, balloon-tipped catheter (such as the Swan-Ganz) into the right side of the heart. [41] The external jugular vein is the vessel of choice for catheter insertion, but the subclavian, femoral, or antecubital veins can be used. [41] Catheter position is determined by the pressure waveform obtained. The pulmonary artery end-diastolic pressure (LVEDP), which is one of the best indicators of left ventricular function [41] It is felt that the PAP readings are more accurate parameters than the central venous pressure because they are more direct and show specific alterations in the left heart hemodynamics. [5]

When the PAP and CVP readings correlate, the PAP will be altered earlier than the CVP. [5] Use of the PAP catheter allows detection of rising pressure very early so that interventions can be instituted to correct the situation. The literature reveals some variability in regard to normal pressure readings: (1) right atrial pressure 3 to 8 mm Hg, (2) right ventricular pressure 20/5 mm Hg, (3) pulmonary artery pressure 25/10 mm Hg, and (4) mean pulmonary artery wedge pressure (reflects left atrial pressure) 5 to 12 mm Hg. [5,26,44] Complications of pulmonary artery catheterization include:[5]

1. Development of cardiac arrhythmias

2. Kinking of the catheter

3. Microemboli

4. Air embolus

5. Lung ischemia if the catheter remains inflated in the wedge position

6. Infection of the catheter site

7. Phlebitis

8. Balloon rupture

CARDIAC CATHETERIZATION

Cardiac catheterization is another type of invasive diagnostic technique. It is utilized to:

1. Obtain multiple pressure measurements in the four heart chambers

2. Determine pulmonary blood flow and cardiac output

3. Obtain samples of blood from the various chambers for analysis of oxygen content, saturation, and tension

4. Inject contrast material for selective angiography to determine the presence and location of obstructive valvular lesions

5. Detect shunts, congenital anomalies, and acquired valvular lesions [4,40]

The sterile procedure takes place in a cardiac catheterization laboratory and takes anywhere from 1 to 3 hours. The client's electrocardiogram is monitored throughout the procedure. [40] There are several studies that may be performed during cardiac catheterization: right heart study, left heart study, coronary arteriography, angiography, and cardiac output. [40]

Right heart catheterization is accomplished by the insertion of a catheter into the antecubital or femoral vein with passage into the inferior or superior vena cava (depending on the point of insertion). The catheter is then advanced into the (1) right atrium, (2) right ventricle, (3) pulmonary artery, and (4) finally wedged in a small distal branch of the pulmonary vasculature. [40] Blood samples and pressure recordings are obtained as the catheter is advanced through each area. Pressure gradients across the valves are also routinely determined to identify any stenosis present and its degree of severity. [40]

Left heart catheterization can be accomplished by three methods:

1. Retrograde catheterization of the aorta is the method of choice; a second catheter is inserted through the femoral or brachial artery and is passed down the ascending aorta, across the aortic valve, and into the left ventricle. Blood samples, pressure readings, and gradients also are taken in the same manner as they are in right heart catheterization.

2. Transseptal puncture is used when stenosis of the aortic valve may necessitate the use of a catheter with a curved tip which is inserted intravenously; the atrial septum must be punctured and the catheter advanced to the left atrium through the mitral valve and into the left ventricle.

3. Direct puncture of the left ventricle is rarely used. [40]

Cardiac Angiography

In coronary arteriography, a catheter is positioned into the coronary arteries and contrast material is injected and recorded cineradiographically so that the blood vessels and the collateral circulation can be visualized and any obstruction can be evaluated. [40] In angiography, the contrast material is injected into the heart chambers to determine (1) chamber size, (2) valvular stenosis, and (3) septal or valvular defects. [40]

Cardiac Output

Cardiac output can be measured by two methods:

1. Fick principle implies that the cardiac output per minute can be determined by measuring the amount of blood that the right ventricle pumps into the lung capillaries within 1 minute (three laboratory measurements are needed: the client's oxygen consumption in milliliters per minute at rest, oxygen content of the arterial blood, and oxygen content of the mixed venous blood taken from the right ventricle or pulmonary artery).

2. With indicator dilution methods the client receives a measured IV injection of dye, arterial blood samples are drawn and the concentration of dye in the blood is determined with special measuring devices. [26] The reading appears as a curve whose size indicates how much blood the heart has pumped out in a given amount of time. [26]

Before cardiac catheterization, the client should be informed that he may feel some unusual sensations during the procedure such as palpitations, warmth, nausea, and headache. The client should be encouraged to report any pain or discomfort to the cardiologist during the procedure. As with all procedures the client should receive a detailed explanation of the procedure, reassurance, and understanding to decrease his level of anxiety. An assessment of the status of the client's pulses distal to the catheterization entry sites should be made prior to and following the procedure. The client remains fasting before the examination and may receive sedation to alleviate anxiety. [40]

Nursing interventions after cardiac catheterization include:

1. Frequent monitoring of vital signs until the client's condition is stable.

2. Apical pulses should be taken.

3. Bed rest should be encouraged for approximately 12 hours depending on the cardiologist.

4. Arterial puncture sites should be checked for bleeding/ hematoma formation (sandbags may be needed to increase pressure to the site).

5. Pulses distal to the punctured vessel should be checked; sudden pain with white, blotchy skin indicates vascular insufficiency and requires immediate medical intervention.

6. Observation for signs of thrombophlebitis (warmth, pain, swelling, and redness) or other systemic complications caused by emboli.

7. Fluids are usually encouraged to prevent dehydration from the dye used during catheterization. [40]

Peripheral, Thoracic, and Abdominal Angiography

Peripheral, thoracic, and abdominal angiography is used to (1) evaluate abnormalities of vascular structure and function, (2) identify mass lesions by vessel displacement and abnormal areas of vascularity, and (3) identify bleeding sites. [40] The femoral artery usually is chosen as the puncture site. Contrast material is injected into the artery through a needle or catheter. As the contrast material is automatically injected, rapid sequence films are taken. All phases of circulation are demonstrated. The client and/or x-ray equipment may be repositioned for special clarifying views. The client should be observed throughout the examination for cardiovascular alterations—blood pressure readings, ECG monitoring, and peripheral pulses. At the conclusion of the examination procedure a pressure dressing is applied and requires frequent observation. [40]

CHAPTER 5

PHYSICAL ASSESSMENT OF THE CARDIOVASCULAR SYSTEM

HISTORICAL DATA IN RELATION TO THE CARDIOVASCULAR SYSTEM

Obtaining the client's historical data is the foundation of the phase of assessment and must be interpreted in view of the other client data collected. The nurse assumes the responsibility for obtaining complete, accurate, and unbiased information during the client interview. The interview provides the nurse with an opportunity to initiate a working and trusting relationship with the client. Historical data related to the cardiovascular system must be interpreted in relation to the other data that has been obtained.

1. Chief complaint

2. History of present illness

3. General health

4. Previous medical/surgical history

5. Past and current therapies

6. Personal history (i. e. , marital status, habits, occupation, education, review of typical day, etc.)

7. Family health history

8. Review of systems (respiratory, circulatory, digestive, musculoskeletal, urinary obstetric and gynecologic, neurologic)

9. Special senses

10. Allergies

Historical data collection is not limited to the initial client contact. Data collection is a continuing process which extends throughout the client-nurse relationship. The initial interview may necessarily be limited so that the client's immediate needs may be met. The source of the historical data obtained (the informant) should be identified, since someone other than the client may be providing or supplementing information, such as family, friends, physicians, other nurses, the client's chart or Kardex.[14,39] All current symptoms or problems (subjective data) mentioned by the client during the interview must be explored in detail. In other words, an analysis of the symptoms takes place. The nurse is interested in obtaining a complete chronology of events in relation to the present illness.

Symptom Analysis

Symptom analysis includes: (1) onset and duration of the symptom, (2) precipitating/predisposing events, (3) characteristics of the pain or discomfort, and (4) related or associated factors.[14,39]

It is important to determine when the symptom first appeared, how long it lasted, and how often it recurs. The client should be encouraged to discuss any precipitating or predisposing events such as the setting (i.e., was the client at home or at work, active or resting, eating or fasting, emotionally upset or relaxed), time of day the symptom occurred and a general description of what took place. The characteristics of any pain should also be explored as to:

1. Location: area where pain begins and any area to which it may radiate.

2. Quality or nature of the pain: Is it burning, gnawing, vise-like, stabbing, squeezing, etc.?

3. Quantity: How many times was the pain experienced and how long did it last, was the pain severe enough to cause the client to stop the activity that he was engaged in, and did the intensity of the pain change?

4. Aggravating factors: What makes the pain feel worse (i.e., eating, drinking, position, activity, seasonal factors)?

5. Alleviating factors: What makes the pain less severe (i.e., medical treatments, position change, activity change)?

6. Related or associated factors: any other symptoms or sensations that are associated with the primary symptom which may occur before, during, or after it.[14,39]

Historical Review of the Cardiovascular System

A historical review of the cardiovascular system should include:

1. Whether or not the client has had a past problem which was related to his heart or blood vessels.

2. Has he ever been told that he had an enlarged heart, murmur, heart attack, or heart failure?

3. Has he ever had an abnormal electrocardiogram, angina pectoris, high cholesterol, hypertension, rheumatic fever, chest pain or discomfort, claudication, dyspnea, edema of the ankles, dizzy or fainting spells, palpitations, unexplained fatigue, coughing during the night, or hemoptysis?[30]

Other screening questions should include: how many pillows does the client use to sleep on at night, does he have nocturia, are his calves tender or edematous, and are varicose veins present? Cardiovascular risk factors have been discussed in Chapter 1 and may be reviewed by the reader. As was mentioned previously, the historical data related to the cardiovascular system must be interpreted in relation to the "total" medical history.

PHYSICAL EXAMINATION OF THE HEART

Physical examination of the heart includes the techniques of inspection, palpation, percussion, and auscultation. If the examiner is right-handed, he should stand to the right of the client during the examination.

Inspection

Inspection involves visual observation of the precordium to determine the effect of ventricular contraction. The apical impulse may be visually located somewhere in the 4th, 5th, or 6th left intercostal space medial to the midclavicular line.[38] The apical impulse may not be visible in many adults; it is located very close to the cardiac apex and can be a useful index of cardiac size. The location of the apical impulse should be described by using the appropriate interspace and the midsternal or midclavicular line (MCL) as reference points. If the heart is enlarged or displaced, the apical impulse may be visible lateral to the MCL. A slight retraction of the intercostal space where the apical impulse is found is a normal finding.[38] However, actual retraction of the rib is an abnormal finding and may be due to pericardial disease. Lift or heave is an abnormal finding found when cardiac action is abnormally forceful especially in the right ventricle when the sternum can be observed to lift with each heartbeat.[38] Slight movement is sometimes referred to as "lift"; a more vigorous movement as "heave." Both terms are often used synonymously to mean the same thing.

Palpation

Palpation is the second technique used in examination of the heart. The examiner's hands should be warm and the client should be comfortable. The apical impulse may not be visible in all adults; however, the cardiac apex often may be located by determining the point of maximum impulse (PMI) using the technique of palpation. This technique should be performed methodically with the client in the supine position if his condition permits. Some examiners prefer to begin palpation at the apex and ascend toward the base of the heart. Others prefer to begin at the second right intercostal space and "inch" their way downward toward the apex. Either technique is acceptable as long as the entire precordium is palpated. The examiner first locates the apical impulse and then proceeds to search for abnormalities such as heaves, thrills, or retractions. A thrill is a palpatory sensation or vibration resulting from the abnormal flow of blood.[28] All findings should be reported in terms of interspace and relation to the midsternal, midclavicular, or axillary lines. The apical impulse produced may be increased in force and duration if the client is experiencing anxiety, anemia, fever, hyperthyroidism, or left ventricular hypertrophy.[28]

Percussion

Percussion is primarily performed to determine the location of the left cardiac border. Percussion is usually performed by percussing in the fourth left intercostal space from the anterior axillary line toward the midline. [38] Some clinicians feel that the actual size of the heart is determined more accurately by chest x-ray. [28]

Auscultation

Auscultation should be performed with the client in at least two positions: sitting and recumbent. The diaphragm of the stethoscope should be checked for cracks before proceeding. Valve closure sounds are best heard in specific locations:

1. Aortic area: in the second right interspace at the sternal border

2. Pulmonic area: second left interspace at the sternal border

3. Tricuspid valve area: near the lower end of the sternum

4. Mitral valve area: at the cardiac apex

The entire precordium should be auscultated in addition to the valve areas mentioned. Valve sounds, murmurs, and other sounds can be detected during the technique of auscultation. A description of the sound auscultated should be made in regard to: (1) intensity or loudness of the sound, (2) quality (i.e.. sharp, dull, snapping), and (3) whether it sounds like a single or split sound. [38]

The first apical heart sound (S1) is usually duller, lower pitched and slightly longer than the second heart sound (S2): the second heart sound is higher in pitch, snappier and shorter than S1. [38]

The technique of auscultation should begin in the aortic area using the diaphragm of the stethoscope because the sounds heard here are of a higher pitch. The second heart sound in

the aortic area (A2) is usually louder than the first heart sound
in the aortic area (A1).* In each area, one should concentrate
initially on the first sound and then on the second sound. Next.
attention should be shifted to the interval between the first
sound and the second sound.

After the aortic area has been auscultated, the examiner
proceeds to the pulmonic area using the same technique. P2
(second heart sound in the pulmonic area) is normally louder
than P1 (first sound in the pulmonic area). Next A2 is compared with P2.

After examining the aortic and pulmonic areas, the examiner
"inches" the stethoscope from the pulmonic area downward to the
lower end of the sternum. In the tricuspid area, the first heart
sound (sometimes referred to as T1) is usually louder than the
second heart sound (T2). In the mitral or apical area, the first
sound (S1) is usually louder than the second beat sound (S2).

If there is a delay in the closure of the valves, a splitting
sound (two distinct components) may be heard. Frequently
splitting of the first heart sound at the apex and the second
heart sound at the base of the heart are heard. A "physiologic
split" of P2 frequently can be heard during deep inspiration in
normal hearts. 10, 38 "Inspiratory splitting of P2" is attributed
to increased venous return to the right ventricle during inspiration which slightly prolongs right ventricular systole and delays
closure of the pulmonic valve. 10 "Expiratory splitting of P2"
is always considered abnormal. A split which does not vary
with respiration is referred to as a fixed split and if the split
is more pronounced on deep expiration. it is called a paradoxical split.38 Both of these splits are abnormal findings.

A third or fourth heart sound also may be heard during cardiac auscultation and occurs during diastole. The third heart
sound (S3) is accepted as being normal in young adults, but is
is considered abnormal in clients over 40 years of age. S3 may
accentuated by placing the client in the left lateral decubitus
position.

---

*The author has elected to use an alternate system of naming
the first and second heart sound in the aortic, pulmonic, and
tricuspid area. This varies from the traditional method. but
is felt that the reader should be aware of alternate methods
sometimes used in the literature. 38, 28, 10

Other third sound features include:

1. It is heard at the apex of the heart.

2. It is low pitched (bell of the stethoscope should be used to hear it).

3. It may become louder with expiration.

4. It occurs early in diastole.

5. It may be more prominent with tachycardia. [38]

The fourth heart sound is heard at the end of the diastolic interval just before systole begins. It may be heard in any location, but it is often heard best at the base of the heart.

A gallop or triple rhythm may be detected. The triple rhythm consists of S1, S2, and a third heart sound of varied origin. [38] This rhythm is best detected at the cardiac apex with the client in the supine position. A determination should be made as to whether the gallop is systolic or diastolic.

Cardiac murmurs are sounds resulting from turbulent blood flow within the heart at the valves or through abnormal openings such as atrial or ventricular septal defects. [38] A bruit is the term reserved for a similar sound which is heard over arteries outside the heart. Murmurs do not necessarily indicate heart disease. The murmur is timed in relation to the first and second heart sounds.

1. Systolic murmurs occur between S1 and S2 and may be referred to as early systolic, midsystolic, holosystolic, or late systolic murmurs.

2. Diastolic murmurs are heard early (immediately after the second sound and fade out in late diastole) or late in diastole (begin near middiastole and become louder as they merge into the first sound). [38]

The murmur should be described by the chest location where the sound is loudest. The location may not correspond to the valve sites due to the transmission of sounds. [38] Erb point (the third left interspace at the sternal border) is frequently called the "secondary aortic area" because aortic valve murmurs are frequently radiated here. Any radiation of the murmur should be described as well as the pitch of the murmur (i.e., low, medium, or high). Other descriptive terms such as blowing, harsh, rumbling, etc. may be used to describe the murmur. The loudness or intensity of a murmur should be recorded according to a six grade system. [38]

Grade I: faintest murmur that can be heard

Grade II: faint, but no problem hearing it

Grade III: soft, but louder than II

Grade IV: loud

Grade V: louder than IV, but not heard if the stethoscope is lifted from the chest

Grade VI: maximum loudness, heard when the stethoscope is lifted from the chest

Figure 12 depicts several types of murmurs as well as their variations in timing, duration and contour.

Another abnormal sound that may be heard during auscultation is the friction rub. This usually is heard when pericarditis is present. The sound usually is not related to systole or diastole and it is typically transient.

PHYSICAL EXAMINATION OF THE PERIPHERAL VASCULAR SYSTEM

Arteries

Inspection is carried out to detect the signs of arterial insufficiency or impairment of the arterial blood flow to the periphery. The signs of arterial insufficiency are (1) pallor, (2) coldness, and (3) nutritional changes (i.e., failure of nail and hair growth on the dorsum of the phalanges, atrophy of the skin and subcutaneous tissues of the finger tips). [27]

A technique to demonstrate arterial insufficiency in the lower limbs is to elevate the legs to 90° with the trunk. The veins and capillaries empty rapidly and pallor develops within a few seconds. When the legs are lowered, color returns slowly and irregularly and the forefoot may develop a deep red color (reactive hyperemia). The rate and degree of color

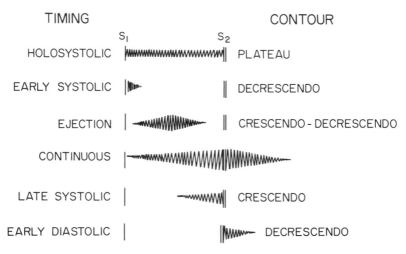

Figure 12. Phonocardiographic characteristic of several
types of murmurs illustrating variations in timing, duration,
and contour. (Reproduced with permission from Anthony, C.
et al. : Pediatric Cardiology — Medical Outline Series.
Garden City, NY: Medical Examination Publishing Co. , Inc. ,
1979, p. 35.)

changes that take place are a clue to the severity of the arterial
insufficiency. If one limb is normal, it can be used as a control. An impairment in arterial blood flow causes a delay in
venous filling. [27] The main arteries to the limb are relatively
normal in young clients suffering from Raynaud disease. However, the small arteries of the fingers constrict when exposed
to a moderate degree of coldness. Fingers become white, cold,
and insensitive. This is followed by cyanosis and painful rubor
from the increased blood flow with recovery. [27]

Visible arterial pulsations of the neck, aorta, and brachial
arteries may also be detected during the technique of inspection.
Palpation is incorporated as an examination technique to determine if there is any change in the pulses or of the temperature.
Normal pulses can be felt in most of the main arteries of the
limbs and neck. Arteries which are easily palpable are the
(1) common carotid, (2) temporal, (3) subclavian, (4) brachial,

(5) radial and ulnar, (6) abdominal aorta, (7) femoral arteries, (8) popliteal, (9) posterior tibial, and (10) dorsalis pedis. Frequently, the posterior tibial and dorsalis pedis arteries cannot be palpated in the elderly client.[27] The volume of pulses can be graded by the following scale.[3, 29, 36]

0   pulse absent

1+   weak

2+   normal

3+   strong

4+   bounding

When there is impaired blood flow to a limb, the <u>temperature</u> is decreased toward the periphery.

<u>Auscultation</u> is performed to detect any systolic bruits over the major arteries. It must be remembered that pressing down on an artery too firmly with the bell of the stethoscope can cause a sound resembling a murmur or bruit. Bruits over the internal carotid, renal, and iliac arteries are most common.[27]

Veins

Venous circulatory impairment may be caused by (1) obstruction to blood flow by thrombosis, phlebitis, or external pressure and by (2) incompetence of the valves in varicose veins. The techniques of <u>inspection</u> and <u>palpation</u> are utilized to detect these processes. The lower limbs should be carefully inspected if the client is on bed rest. Reliable signs of <u>venous thrombosis</u> are increased warmth, swelling, duskiness of the skin of the calf, pitting edema of the ankle on the affected side, and dilatation of the small veins over the tibia of one leg.[27] If the affected limb is elevated, the dilated veins do not empty normally. Gentle palpation of the calf of the affected limb may elicit tenderness and one calf may be larger than the other.[27] Homan sign (forceful dorsiflexion of the foot) may or may not be positive. There is some disagreement as to whether this test should be performed by the examiner since the possibility exists that a thrombus may be dislodged by the maneuver.[27]

<u>Varicose veins</u> can be detected by having the client stand during the technique of inspection and palpation. Maximal

dilatation often is seen in the area of the inner side of the calf or above the ankle.[27] The Trendelenburg test may be used to demonstrate competence of valves. This test requires empty-ing the leg veins by elevation of the limb; the long saphenous vein is then compressed by a light tourniquet at the saphenous opening and the client stands.[27] If the vein fills from below, the valves in the communicating veins are incompetent. A venogram may be necessary to demonstrate the exact extent of the incompetence.

Jugular Veins

A general estimate of venous return and filling volume can be made by observing the jugular veins.[28] The jugular veins may be examined with the client in the supine position or with the client's trunk elevated to a 45° angle. Client preparation includes: (1) removal of clothing from the neck and upper thorax, (2) head and neck comfortably positioned on a pillow, and (3) client's neck turned slightly away from the side being observed.[28] Normally, no jugular pulsations are visible when the client is in a sitting position.[28] When the client is supine, the venous pulse becomes evident. The venous pulse consists of three positive components (i.e., a, c, and v waves) and two negative slopes (i.e., x and y descents).[28]

The "a" wave is produced by atrial contraction and it occurs just before S1. The "c" wave is produced by two simul-taneous events: (1) the impact of the adjacent carotid artery pulsation and (2) retrograde transmission of a pulse wave.[28] This wave occurs at the end of S1. The "v" wave is sometimes referred to as the passive filling wave and it reaches its peak during late ventricular diastole. An increased volume in the vena cava and the right atrium leads to a pressure increase which is reflected in the jugular veins.[28] The "x" descent which follows the c wave is produced by the downward displace-ment of the base of the ventricles and the tricuspid valve during ventricular contraction and atrial filling.[28] The "y" descent follows the v wave and is produced by the opening of the tricus-pid valve and the rapid flow of blood from the right atrium to the right ventricle that follows.[28]

Abnormally enlarged a waves may be seen in conditions such as: tricuspid valve stenosis; right ventricular enlargement due to severe pulmonary stenosis or pulmonary hypertension; complete AV block; and ventricular tachycardia. The negative x slope may become obliterated or replaced by the positive c and v waves when the tricuspid valve is insufficient and blood regurgitates from the right ventricle to the right atrium during ventricular systole. The enlarged c-v wave then resembles an exaggerated arterial pulsation.[28] The y descent would be slow if tricuspid stenosis were present due to the obstruction to right atrial emptying.[28]

Jugular Venous Pressure

When a client is examined with the thorax at a 45° angle elevation, the venous pulses should ascend no more than a few millimeters above the clavicle.[28] If the venous pressure is markedly elevated, the neck veins may be distended up to the angle of the jaw. Venous pressure may be estimated by measuring the distance that the veins are distended above the manubrium sterni.[28] The position of the client should be recorded along with the level to which the distention is observed. Venous pressure elevations may be seen in (1) congestive heart failure, (2) constrictive pericarditis, or (3) obstruction of the superior vena cava.

CHAPTER 6

HUMAN SEXUALITY IN RELATION TO CARDIOVASCULAR DISEASE

Sexuality is a quality of being human. Although a person's sex is genetically determined, sexuality is also influenced by the psychosocial environment in which the person lives and interacts. [13] Therefore, it can be said that heredity and learning interact to produce a given type of sexuality. [15] Fonseca states that: "Man's sexuality is intrinsic to his being and colors his thoughts, ideas, social interactions, physical well-being, and his ability not only to reproduce but to nurture his offspring." [13] Although human sexuality is more than the physical sex act, this chapter will focus on the topic of sex and the cardiac client, since this aspect has often been neglected in the acute care setting in years past.

During recent years, studies have been carried out to determine the physiologic effects of sexual intercourse. Studies by Masters and Johnson (1966) conducted in laboratory settings with young, healthy subjects suggest that intercourse is associated with marked cardiovascular fluctuations (i.e., tachycardia, blood pressure elevation, and respiratory rate increases). [43] These fluctuations are dramatic but brief and drop to normal levels a few minutes after orgasm. The investigators Hellerstein and Friedman concluded from their studies that the physiologic cost of sexual intercourse for the middle-aged, middle-class, long-married man was modest. [43]

The physician and the nurse both bear the responsibility of counseling the cardiac client. Planned, structured counseling sessions can help to alleviate the fear, ignorance, and misinformation which increase the client's level of anxiety and frustration. Moore et al. polled more than 30 people to determine which questions were most frequently asked by cardiac clients. The clients most frequently asked (1) Would sexual intercourse ever be possible again? (2) If so, how soon and how often? (3) How dangerous was the exertion required? (4) Do cardiac drugs affect sexual activity? (5) How would the sex partner react to the problem? and (6) How could the cardiac client discuss the subject of sex with his partner?[31]

Although the physician should decide when the client may resume sexual activity, many clients are able to resume their previous sexual life in about 4 to 5 weeks after their heart attack.[31] There is controversy in the literature regarding the time when sexual activity can be resumed. Rule states that sexual activity may be resumed in about 3 months post-MI.[35] "When" sexual activity can resume is a highly individualized matter. When the client has been able to return to his/her "usual" activities and when the laboratory tests and the electrocardiogram are essentially normal, the physician will usually inform the client that sexual activity may be resumed.

Some authorities suggest that the client's sexual history be collected as a basis for counseling. The sexual history assists the interviewer in identifying the client's needs, concerns, problems, and misconceptions; and in defining areas for education, counseling, and reassurances.[11] The client has an opportunity to verbalize questions and feelings. The data obtained should assist the nurse in developing a more comprehensive nursing care plan. Nurses who are not comfortable dealing with sexual problems should refer clients to other appropriate health members or agencies for assistance.

Some practical approaches to performing a sexual assessment found in current nursing literature include: (1) client preparation--informing the client that some personal questions may be asked during the health history to identify any problems that may need resolution, (2) allow the client not to answer the question if it is anxiety producing, (3) use a vocabulary that the client can understand, (4) questions should progress from topics that are easier to discuss to those that are more difficult, (5) use matter-of-fact approach, (6) a suggested sequence of topics might be birth and reproduction, previous attitudes or feelings regarding childbirth, coitus, nocturnal emissions, menstruation, masturbation, premarital-extramarital affairs, difficulties in coitus, sex dreams, and client questions.[11,24] It is important to provide privacy during the interview and ensure confidentiality. The nurse should allow adequate time for the client to discuss and explore needs, attitudes, feelings, values, expectations, practices, anxieties, fears, and other problems.[11] Counseling sessions may then be planned to resolve identified problems.

Occasionally physicians object to having the nurse perform a sexual assessment on their client. This is a matter which should be clarified with the physician in charge of the client's care. Most authorities agree that the sex partner of the client with a cardiac condition should be invited to attend counseling sessions designed to teach the client guidelines to minimize cardiac work load during sexual intercourse. This should be determined on an individual basis; separate sessions may be more helpful.

The following are suggested guidelines for the cardiac client. [17, 31]

1. Sexual intercourse resumed in familiar surroundings is less stressful.

2. Extremes in room temperature add stress.

3. Foreplay is desirable since it prepares the heart gradually for intercourse.

4. The position for intercourse should be comfortable and permit unrestricted breathing (the cardiac-on-top position results in sustained isometric arm and shoulder contraction which elevates the central aortic pressure and is therefore undesirable; acceptable positions include: side-lying, back-lying, with the cardiac on the bottom, or with the cardiac seated on a broad armless chair with feet flat on the floor.)

5. Anal intercourse should be avoided since it adds more stress to the heart.

6. Rest before intercourse may be helpful (some find morning an ideal time).

7. Intercourse should be postponed for approximately 3 hours after a heavy meal or drinking, or if the client is tense or tired.

8. Extramarital affairs may be more stressful for the heart.

9. If chest pain occurs during intercourse, the physician may prescribe a medication such as nitroglycerin or isosorbide dinitrate (Isordil).

10. Masturbation may or may not require more energy expenditure than intercourse and the client should discuss this with his physician.

The client should be taught the danger signs that should be reported to his physician promptly. These include: shortness of breath, increasing heart rate or palpitations for longer than 15 minutes after intercourse, chest pain, extreme fatigue the day after intercourse, or sleeplessness after intercourse.[31]

The counseling sessions should assist in decreasing the level of anxiety in both the client and the spouse, so that they may return to their previous level of sexual activity.

REVIEW QUESTIONS TO PART II

1. Does the apex of the heart point upward or downward? To the right or to the left?

2. Describe the following structures of the heart:

   Pericardium   Coronary blood supply

   Heart wall   Cardiac muscle

   Heart chambers   Conduction system

   Heart valves

3. What cardiac events cause the appearance of the heart sounds?

4. Discuss the following properties of cardiac muscle which are essential for regulation of heart rate and rhythm:

   Rhythmicity   Contractility

   Irritability   Automaticity

   Refractoriness   Extensibility

   Conductivity

5. Describe the function of the following:

   Autonomic nervous system

   Sinoatrial node

   Atrioventricular

   Bundle of His-Purkinje system

6. Blood vessels are composed of three layers. Name them.

7. Which blood vessels have the thickest walls?

8. Which blood vessels have the thinnest walls?

9. How do veins differ from arteries in their structure?

10. Describe the following noninvasive diagnostic techniques:

Echocardiogram   Exercise testing

Phonocardiogram   Electrocardiogram

11. List the 12 leads recorded in a standard ECG.

12. Define the following:

Bipolar leads

Unipolar leads

Einthoven triangle

P wave

QRS complex

ST segment

T Wave

13. Which cardiac enzymes occur in, and are released by, cardiac tissue?

14. Which cardiac enzyme rises and falls faster than the other cardiac enzymes?

15. CPK can be fractioned into three isoenzymes. Name them.

16. Of the enzymes named in question 13, which enzyme is the least specific for cardiac disease?

17. Define the following:

    CVP   Erb point

    PAP   Physiological split

    Apical impulse   Gallop rhythm

    Lift or heave   Murmur

    Bruit

18. What diagnostic information can be obtained from performing a cardiac catheterization?

19. Describe the structures through which the catheter passes when right heart catheterization is performed.

20. Name the three methods that may be utilized to accomplish left heart catheterization.

21. What are the two methods by which cardiac output can be measured?

22. Identify at least six nursing interventions that should be carried out after cardiac catheterization.

23. For what purposes would peripheral, thoracic and abdominal angiography be carried out?

24. Describe the screening questions that should be included in a historical review of the cardiovascular system.

25. Explain the techniques of inspection, palpation, percussion, and auscultation in relation to physical examination of the heart.

26. What are the signs of arterial insufficiency?

27. Using a grading scale of 0 to 4+, what significance would a 2+ have in relation to pulse volume?

28. What are three conditions in which an increase in jugular venous pressure may be seen?

29. Describe some practical approaches to performing a sexual assessment on a client experiencing cardiovascular problems.

30. Name the danger signs during or following intercourse that the client should report to his physician.

REFERENCES TO PART II

1. Adams, N., Beaumont, W., Vasquez, A., Krezmien, L., Blackwell, C.: Reducing the Perils of Intracardiac Monitoring. Nursing 76 (April 1976): 66-74.

2. Andreoli, K. G. et al.: Comprehensive Cardiac Care. St. Louis: C. V. Mosby Co., 1968.

3. Bates, B.: A Guide to Physical Examination. Philadelphia: J. B. Lippincott Co., 1974, pp. 218-225, 1979.

4. Beyers, M. and Dudas, S.: The Clinical Practice of Medical-Surgical Nursing. Boston: Little, Brown and Company, 1977.

5. Bologinini, V.: The Swan-Ganz Pulmonary Artery Catheter: Implications For Nursing. Heart Lung 3 (November-December 1974): 976-981.

6. Browning M. and Lewis, E. (Eds.): Human Sexuality: Nursing Implications. New York: American Journal of Nursing Co., 1973.

7. Conover, M. H. and Zalis, E. G.: Understanding Electrocardiography. St. Louis: C. V. Mosby Co., 1976.

8. Conover, M. H.: Cardiac Arrhythmias. 2nd Ed., St. Louis: C. V. Mosby Co., 1978.

9. Daly, J., Ziegler, B., Dudrick, S.: Central Venous Catheterization. Am J Nurs 75 (May 1975): 820-824.

10. DeGowin, E. and DeGowin, R.: Bedside Diagnostic Evaluation. 2nd Ed. New York: Macmillan Co., 1969, pp. 316-435.

11. Elder, M.S.: The Unmet Challenge-Nurse Counseling on Sexuality. In Browning, M. and Lewis, E. (Eds.): Human Sexuality: Nursing Implications. New York: American Journal of Nursing Co., 1973, pp. 39-46.

12. Fisher, R. E.: Measuring Central Venous Pressure. Nursing 79 (October 1979): 74-78.

13. Fonseca, J.: Sexuality--A Quality of Being Human. In Browning, M. and Lewis, E. (Eds.): Human Sexuality: Nursing Implications. New York: American Journal of Nursing Co., 1973, pp. 1, 2.

14. Gillies, D. A. and Alyn, I.: Patient Assessment and Management by the Nurse Practitioner. Philadelphia: W.B. Saunders Co., 1976.

15. Goldstein, B.: Human Sexuality. New York: McGraw-Hill Book Co., 1976.

16. Gowen, F.: Interpretation of Central Venous Pressure. Surg Clin N Am 53 (June 1973): 649. Cited by Brenda Haughey: C.V.P. Lines: Monitoring and Maintaining. Am J Nurs 78 (April 1978): 637.

17. Green, R. (Ed.): Human Sexuality. Baltimore: Williams & Wilkins Co., 1975.

18. Guyton, A.: Textbook of Medical Physiology. 5th Ed., Philadelphia: W.B. Saunders Co., 1976.

19. Haughey, B.: C.V.P. Lines: Monitoring and Maintaining. Am J Nurs 78 (April 1978): 635-638.

20. Henrick, A. and Stephanides, L.: Common Diagnostic Uses of Echocardiography. Cardiovasc Nurs 14 (September-October 1978): 21-25.

21. Hobson, L.: Examination of the Patient. New York: McGraw-Hill Book Co., 1975.

22. Hudak, C., Lohr, T., Gallo, B.: Critical Care Nursing. 2nd Ed., Philadelphia: J.B. Lippincott Co., 1977.

23. Jacob S. and Francone, C.: Structure and Function in Man. Philadelphia: W.B. Saunders Co., 1970, 1978.

24. Krozy, R.: Becoming Comfortable with Sexual Assessment. Am J Nurs 78 (June 1978): 1036-1038.

25. Lamb, J.: Intra-Arterial Monitoring. Nursing 77 (November 1977): 65-71.

26. Luckmann, J. and Sorensen, K.: Medical-Surgical Nursing, A Psychophysiologic Approach. Philadelphia: W. B. Saunders Co., 1974, 1980.

27. Macleod, J. (Ed.): Clinical Examination. New York: Churchhill Livingstone, 1976, pp. 103-153.

28. Malasanos, L., Barkauskas, V., Moss, M., Stoltenberg-Allen, K.: Health Assessment. St. Louis: C. V. Mosby Co., 1977, pp. 216-231.

29. Miller, B. and Keane, C.: Encyclopedia and Dictionary of Medicine, Nursing and Allied Health. 2nd Ed., Philadelphia: W. B. Saunders Co., 1978, pp. 316, 200.

30. Miller, K.: Assessing Peripheral Perfusion. Am J Nurs 78 (October 1978): 1673-1674.

31. Moore, K., Folk-Lighty, M., Nolan, M. J.: The Joy of Sex After a Heart Attack. Nursing 77 (June 1977): 53-55.

32. Nanda, N. C.: Clinical Applications of Echocardiography. Mod Conc Cardiovasc Dis 45 (November 1976): 135-138.

33. Rapaport, E.: Serum Enzymes and Isoenzymes in the Diagnosis of Acute Myocardial Infarction. Part II: Isoenzymes. Mod Conc Cardiovasc Dis 46 (October 1977): 47-50.

34. Ross, J. and O'Rourke, R.: Understanding the Heart and Its Diseases. New York: McGraw-Hill Book Co., 1976.

35. Rule, D.: The Road Back Begins in the C. C. U. Nursing 77 (March 1977): pp. 48-51.

36. Sauve', M. J. and Pecherer, A.: Concepts and Skills in Physical Assessment. Philadelphia: W. B. Saunders Co., 1977, pp. 89-107, 327-340.

37. Scheer, E.: Enzymatic Changes and Myocardial Infarction: A Nursing Update. Cardiovasc Nurs 14 (March-April 1978): 5-8.

38. Sherman, J. and Field, S.: Guide to Patient Evaluation. Garden City, NY: Medical Examination Publishing Co., Inc., 1974, pp. 131-151.

39. Silverman, M.: Examination of the Heart. Part I: The Clinical History. American Heart Association, Inc., 1975.

40. Skydell, B. and Crowder, A.: Diagnostic Procedures. Boston: Little, Brown and Co., 1975, pp. 127-133.

41. Smith, R. N.: Invasive Pressure Monitoring. Am J Nurs 78 (September 1978): 1514-1521.

42. Strong, A. B.: Caring For Cardiac Catheterization Patients. Nursing 77 (November 1977): 60-64.

43. Wagner, N.: Sexual Activity and the Cardiac Patient. In Green, R. (Ed.): Human Sexuality. Williams & Wilkins Co., 1975, pp. 172-179.

44. Woods, S.: Monitoring Pulmonary Artery Pressures. Am J Nurs 76 (Nov 1976): 1765-1771.

PART III

SPECIFIC ALTERATIONS IN THE CARDIOVASCULAR SYSTEM

INTRODUCTION

The American Heart Association has identified some of the major diseases of the cardiovascular system which include: hypertension, atherosclerosis, myocardial infarction, cerebral vascular accident, congestive heart failure, rheumatic heart disease, and congenital defects. These, as well as several other common cardiovascular alterations, are presented in this part of the text in alphabetical order rather than in the order of their frequency of occurrence for the convenience of the reader. General categories of cardiovascular pathology included are:

Pump failure (heart muscle): congestive heart failure (right and left ventricular failure)

Common disturbances of rate and/or rhythm: arrhythmias

Developmental (congenital) heart pathology: aortic coarctation

Valvular alterations: rheumatic heart disease

Vascular alterations: aneurysms, angina pectoris, arteriosclerosis-atherosclerosis, Buerger disease, cerebral vascular accident, hypertension, myocardial infarction, pulmonary embolism, Raynaud disease, thrombophlebitis

Each chapter begins with a "description" of the cardiovascular alteration being discussed. A definition as well as a brief description of the pathophysiology involved in the alteration is presented. Classifications are included in this section, as appropriate, for the alteration being discussed.

71

The "etiology" or cause of the alteration or disease process is discussed. If the exact etiology is unknown, the theories of causation which are being explored are presented.

"Assessment" data presented is specific to the alteration being discussed. Historical data collection, findings obtained from physical examination, and diagnostic examinations are included under this heading. The client's symptoms are referred to as "subjective data." Subjective data are obtained from the client or the client's "significant other" (wife, relative, friend). Signs of the alteration or objective findings are referred to as "objective data." These data are obtained by the nurse, physician, and other health team members. Diagnostic tests and their results are included under this section.

General "client care goals" are presented for each cardiovascular alteration presented. These goals are intentionally presented in broad or general terms and it is intended that they serve only as possibilities. It is expected that in clinical practice, specific behavioral goals should be developed individually for each person. Ideally, goal-setting should be a collaborative process which involves the client, the nurse, the physician, and other health team members. The process of goal-setting offers an excellent opportunity for the nurse and other health team members to determine what the client's expectations are in relation to his illness. Stated goals should be realistic and attainable. Specific criteria should be established to determine whether the established goal was indeed realized.

Nursing and medically prescribed interventions for each alteration are described. Interventions determine what will be done to resolve a client's problem or need and are directed toward the accomplishment of established client-care goals. Nursing interventions may be categorized as: assistive, hygienic, rehabilitative, supportive, preventative, observational, or educational. Interventions specific to the cardiovascular alteration are presented in this section. In clinical practice, interventions should be directed to meet the needs of the "total" person.

Complications are included as the last topic for each alteration in the format.

CHAPTER 7

ANEURYSMS

LEARNING OBJECTIVES

Study of this chapter will enable the reader to:

1. Name the classifications of arterial aneurysms

2. Discuss the etiology and predisposing factors favoring the development of aneurysms

3. Describe the subjective data in relation to thoracic and abdominal aneurysms

4. Describe common physical assessment findings that might be expected in abdominal aneurysm

5. Compare the various diagnostic tests available when aneurysm is suspected

6. Plan nursing interventions for the preoperative, intraoperative and postoperative periods

7. Predict possible complications for the client with an aneurysm

DESCRIPTION

An arterial aneurysm is an abnormal dilatation of the wall of an artery. Aneurysms may be singular or multiple and they may be classified as saccular, fusiform, or dissecting.[3, 4]

A saccular aneurysm involves only a part of the circumference of the artery and is caused by localized stretching of the medial layer.[3, 10]

73

A fusiform aneurysm involves the entire circumference of the arterial wall, with tapering at both ends resembling a spindle. [3,10]

A dissecting aneurysm occurs when the blood is forced between the layers of the arterial wall; it may be caused by a degenerative defect in the tunica media. [3,10]

The incidence of aneurysm is higher among older men than women and mortality is high if the aneurysm is not corrected surgically. [3] Spontaneous rupture of the aneurysm is the major cause of death. [3]

ETIOLOGY

The major cause of aneurysm is thought to be arteriosclerosis. [3,5] Syphilis, infections within and around the vessel, trauma, and congenital defects also may predispose to the development of aneurysms. [3] Hypertension and coarctation accelerate the other predisposing factors. [11] It has been said that pregnancy contributes to histochemical changes in the aorta that weaken it. [11]

ASSESSMENT SPECIFIC TO THE ALTERATION

Subjective data (symptoms) and objective data (signs) will be variable according to the location and size of the lesion. It is not unusual for an aneurysm to be asymptomatic and it may be found coincidentally during a routine physical examination or chest x-ray.

THORACIC ANEURYSMS

The aortic arch is the most commonly involved and the aneurysm may be saccular or fusiform.

Subjective Data

There may be no symptoms. When symptoms are present, the client frequently complains of retrosternal pain which radiates to the left scapula, the left shoulder, or left side of the neck. [4] If the aneurysm compresses the left main bronchus or left recurrent laryngeal nerve against the trachea, the client may also complain of a brassy cough and hoarseness. [4] The client may complain of dysphagia if pressure is exerted on the esophagus. [5]

Objective Data

An aneurysm located near the origin of the left subclavian artery may cause a delay of the pulse wave to the left arm with a reduction of more than 20 mm in arterial pressure in that arm; this causes a palpable decrease in pulse volume. [4] If the aneurysm pushes down on the left main bronchus, a tracheal tug may be perceived while palpating the trachea. [4] Pressure on the superior vena cava will cause physical findings such as edema of the neck and arms and/or distended neck veins. [5] The diagnosis is usually confirmed by chest x-ray and aortography and sometimes ultrasonic studies. [5]

ABDOMINAL ANEURYSM

Approximately 80% of the aortic aneurysms are: (1) in the distal aorta, (2) arteriosclerotic in origin, and (3) fusiform in shape. [5] The incidence of abdominal aneurysm is higher in men than in women (4:1 ratio). [9]

Subjective Data

Aneurysms of the abdominal aorta may be asymptomatic. If pain is present, it varies from mild midabdominal or lumbar discomfort to severe constant or intermittent abdominal and back pain. [5] Some clients complain of pain in the lumbar region radiating into the flank or groin. Other complaints may include dull, steady epigastric pain, a sense of fullness after meals, and even nausea and vomiting. [9] If the iliac and femoral arteries have atherosclerotic involvement, the client may complain of claudication and other symptoms of arterial ischemia or occlusion. [9]

Objective Data

Eighty percent of all abdominal aneurysms are palpable. [9] A pulsating mid- and upper-abdominal mass may be discovered on a routine physical examination. [5] A bruit may be heard over the aneurysm. [4] An x-ray showing the lateral lumbar spine may reveal calcification of the wall of the aneurysm. [9] Other findings may be due to cardiac, renal, pulmonary, or distal peripheral obliterative vascular disease not uncommon in clients of this age group. [5]

Diagnostic Tests

Ultrasound examination may be used to determine the size of the aneurysm. Aortography has been utilized to determine the condition of the vessels distal to the aneurysm, where the lower end of the graft will be anastomosed.[9] A comprehensive preoperative clinical assessment includes:[9]

Renal function tests (BUN, creatinine, electrolytes)

Liver function tests

Routine hematology

Cardiology consultation

Pulmonary function tests

Blood gases

An arteriogram

The arteriogram is done to determine:

1. If the renal arteries are involved

2. The condition of arteries distal to the aneurysm

3. The significance of the inferior mesenteric blood flow to the bowel [8, 9]

At present, it is felt that computed tomography (CT) is the best method of assessing abdominal aortic aneurysms. CT has accurately demonstrated the anatomy of the aneurysm. It has been possible to identify those aneurysms whose walls are extremely thin and those that have leaked.[2] It is hoped that in the future, it will be possible to identify aneurysms that are at risk of rupture.[2] The cost of the CT equipment, however, may limit its availability for widespread use in certain areas.

CLIENT CARE GOALS

1. Progression of the alteration will be slowed or halted through prompt diagnosis and interventions.

2. There will be relief of subjective complaints, i.e., pain, cough, hoarseness, dysphagia, edema of the neck, arms, etc.

3. Postoperative complications will be prevented.

4. Hypertensive control and inotropic blockage must be maintained when the client returns home.

5. The client's adaptive processes will be facilitated during all phases of the illness.

INTERVENTIONS: THORACIC ANEURYSMS

Aneurysms of the ascending, transverse, and descending thoracic aorta are treated by means of surgical intervention with the use of some type of total cardiopulmonary bypass. Preoperative and postoperative care of the client is similar to care of the client having heart surgery. 10

Preoperative Period

The client should receive an adequate explanation of all procedures to take place preoperatively, intraoperatively and postoperatively. The physician should explain why the operation should be done, what will be done surgically, and what the expected outcomes are. The nurse who is responsible for the client's care should be present during the physician's explanation, so that the physician's teaching can be reinforced and contradictory statements can be avoided. The client understandably will be anxious and apprehensive and will need a great deal of emotional support from the nurse, family, physician, and clergyman. False reassurances of the prognosis should be avoided. The nurse should obtain some basic data preoperatively regarding the activity level of the client--this will serve as a useful guide postoperatively. 10

Intraoperative Period

In ideal hospital situations, extracorporeal circulation is used during the corrective surgery. Catheters are inserted into the superior and inferior vena cavae for the passage of venous blood flow; another catheter is inserted into the common femoral artery so that oxygenated blood will be returned to the systemic circulation.[10] Ascending thoracic aneurysms are approached through a sternal-splitting incision.[11] The aneurysm is then resected and replaced with a Teflon or Dacron prosthesis.[10] The specific operative procedure can be found in any surgical text.

Postoperative Period

The client will need constant observation for several days in a cardiac recovery room or intensive care unit (ICU). Oxygen, inhalation therapy equipment, and intermittent positive pressure machines may be used: this varies with the individual physician. Other equipment that should be readily available includes: chest suction apparatus, thoracentesis set, emergency medications and other equipment for cardiopulmonary resuscitation, infusion poles, sphygmomanometer stethoscope, suction equipment, and equipment to apply external heat or maintain hypothermia if hypothermia was utilized during surgery.[10] Since the mortality is highest during the first 48 hours, the nurse must be alert for any complications such as hemorrhage, hypotension, fibrillation, arrhythmias, sudden chest pain, and pulmonary edema.[10] The client usually is maintained on continuous respiratory support for a brief period after surgery. This increases the efficiency of breathing and minimizes the complications of hypoxia.[10] The ECG is monitored continuously. CVP and vital signs are monitored and recorded at least every 15 minutes. The patency of the chest tubes and the amount and color of the drainage in the chest bottles are monitored and recorded on an hourly basis. As with any surgical procedure, dressings are inspected frequently for blood. Vitamin K preparations and protamine sulfate may be needed to counteract any bleeding due to the heparin received during surgery.[10] A Foley catheter may be inserted and the urine is collected hourly and checked for specific gravity, color, and amount. Hourly output should not be less than 15 to 30 ml.[10] Electrolytes should be monitored. Narcotics may be prescribed to relieve pain. The client should be encouraged to cough and deep breathe while the incision is splinted. [10] Chest tubes may be removed in 2 to 3 days postoperatively depending on the client's condition and physicians preference. Arm and leg exercises should be instituted while the client is on bed rest. The nurse should be alert for changes in the client's behavior; depression, disorientation, panic and hallucinations are not unusual after cardiac surgery. [10] The time of ambulation varies with the client's progress and condition, as well as with the procedure performed.

INTERVENTIONS: ABDOMINAL ANEURYSM

Medical and surgical cardiac teams are required for effective interventions. The client is placed in ICU for the purpose of controlling blood pressure and instituting negative inotropic therapy before surgical intervention. [11] Surgical excision of the aneurysm and grafting is the treatment of choice except when the lesion is very small and asymptomatic or when the client's general condition is so poor that the surgical risk is greater than the risk of rupture. [5] Despite advances in the operative technique, the operation remains hazardous. [11] Persistent hemorrhage is the most common cause of operative death. [11] Extracorporeal perfusion usually is not necessary, since arterial flow to the lower extremities can be interrupted safely for the length of time needed to complete the operation. [10]

Preoperative Period

The nurse obtains baseline data on the client's physical status (i.e., vital signs, character of peripheral pulses, breath sounds, and review of all other systems). [9] The client's readiness to learn about his surgery should be assessed and a plan should be developed to teach the client and family about the procedures to come. Hopefully, the explanations and psychosocial support given by the nurse will assist in reducing their anxiety. The nurse reviews and evaluates all laboratory values, sees that the client is correctly prepared for surgery, and checks to see that proper permission has been obtained. [9] The nurse should arrange for a visit from the clergyman if the client so desires. The client's weight should be obtained preoperatively. An IV and a Foley catheter may be inserted before surgery. An arterial line and central venous pressure line may also be inserted by the physician. Some physicians insert a pulmonary artery catheter to obtain baseline information and to allow for continuous monitoring of the pulmonary artery pressure (PAP) and the pulmonary artery wedge pressure (PAWP). [9] A nasogastric tube also may be inserted.

Postoperative Period

CVP, heart rate, blood pressure and temperature must be continuously monitored. The client's abdominal girth should be measured and recorded every 2 hours to detect any internal bleeding. [9] An accurate record of intake and output is essential. Urine output is measured every hour; if output is below 30 ml/hr the physician should be informed. Specific gravity of the urine should be checked every 3 to 4 hours; if the client is hypovolemic, the specific gravity will be greater than 1.030. [9] Pulses (i.e., popliteal, pedal, and posterior tibial) as well as temperature, color, and movement of extremities should be assessed hourly. [9] Decreased or absent pulses and cool, mottled extremities may indicate occlusion of the graft. [9] The ECG should be monitored for signs of ventricular irritability such as (1) premature ventricular contractions, (2) inverted T waves, or (3) ST depression or elevation. [9] A neurologic assessment should be performed (i.e., pupil size, response to light, ability to move extremities, quality of hand grasps, and orientation). [9] Frequent respiratory assessments should be done. After the client is extubated, he should be encouraged to cough and deep breathe to prevent respiratory complications. The nurse should routinely check the patency and position of the nasogastric tube. At least once each shift, the color and amount of the drainage, and the results of the guaiac test for blood should be recorded. Ambulation varies with the client's condition and the physician's preference: usually the client is up by the second day and walks with assistance. Sitting should be avoided for the first week to prevent unnecessary pressure on the graft. [9] Routine nursing comfort measures also are instituted. Discharge planning should include teaching the client about his activity schedule, breathing exercises, diet, rest, importance of medical follow-up, and arrangements for a visiting nurse or other homemaker services if necessary.

COMPLICATIONS

Complications include hemorrhage, renal failure, embolization, occlusion of the graft, heart failure, respiratory complications, paralytic ileus and distention, and thrombophlebitis. [9, 10]

REVIEW QUESTIONS

1. Define the term "aneurysm."

2. Name the three classifications of arterial aneurysms.

3. What is the major cause of aneurysms?

4. What other alterations or conditions may predispose one to the development of aneurysms?

5. Are symptoms always present when the client has a thoracic aneurysm? An abdominal aneurysm?

6. Discuss the explanations that a client undergoing repair of an aneurysm should have regarding the preoperative and postoperative periods.

7. Describe nursing interventions during the postoperative period for the client in question 6.

8. List the complications possible when the client has an aneurysm.

REFERENCES

1. Armington, S. C. and Creighton, H.: Nursing of People With Cardiovascular Problems. Boston: Little, Brown and Co., 1971, pp. 262-266.

2. Young, A.E. et al: Assessment of Abdominal Aortic Aneurysms by Computed Tomography. Br Med J (Mar 15, 1980):765.

3. Beyers, M. and Dudas, S.: The Clinical Practice of Medical-Surgical Nursing. Boston: Little, Brown and Co., 1977, pp. 399-401.

4. De Gowin, E. and De Gowin, R.: Bedside Diagnostic Evaluation. 2nd Ed., New York: Macmillan Co., 1969, pp. 424-427.

5. Erskine, J.: Blood Vessels and Lymphatics. In Krupp, M.A. and Chatton, M.J.: Current Medical Diagnosis and Treatment. Los Altos, Calif.: Lange Medical Publications, 1976, pp. 243-247.

6. Gomes, M. and Hufnagel, C.: CT Scanning: A New Method for the Diagnosis of Abdominal Aortic Aneurysms. J Cardiovasc Surg 20, 1979: 511-516.

7. Harvey, A. M. et al.: The Principles and Practice of Medicine. 18th Ed., New York: Appleton-Century-Crofts, 1972, pp. 362-369.

8. Kadir, S. et al.: Tender Pulsatile Abdominal Mass. Arch Surg 115 (May 1980): 631-633.

9. Long, G. D'Onofrio: Managing the Patient with Abdominal Aortic Aneurysm. Nursing 78 (August 1978) 20-27.

10. Shafer, K. et al.: Medical-Surgical Nursing. 6th Ed. St. Louis: C. V. Mosby Co., 1975 pp. 363-371 388-391.

11. Webb, W. R. et al.: Management of Acute Dissections of the Aorta. Heart Lung 9 (March/April 1980): 284-288.

CHAPTER 8

ANGINA PECTORIS

LEARNING OBJECTIVES

Study of this chapter will enable the reader to:

1. Recognize that there are several types of angina

2. Discuss the theories in relation to the etiology of angina pectoris

3. Describe factors to be included in the assessment of the client's pain/discomfort

4. Cite common findings: subjective (symptoms) and objective data (signs) of the client experiencing angina

5. Explain the diagnostic examinations that can be utilized to determine the basis of the client's symptoms

6. Formulate a nursing plan to educate the client in relation to this alteration

7. Discuss antianginal agents: action, side effects, and precautions

8. State possible complications

DESCRIPTION

Angina pectoris may be described as an alteration in which there is acute chest pain resulting from an imbalance between myocardial oxygen supply and myocardial demand or consumption.[12,18] Angina pectoris occurs more frequently in men than in women and in older, rather than younger people. It is often referred to as a "symptom" of an underlying disease of the arteries, rather than a disease entity in itself.[18]

Several types of angina are recognized:

1. Stable angina

2. Unstable angina (sometimes called preinfarction angina, acute coronary insufficiency, crescendo angina, and intermediate syndrome)

3. Variant angina (Printzmetal angina) [3, 5, 10]

   The quality of the pain may vary from client to client; however, the individual generally experiences the same type of pain during each episode of angina.[12] Equilibrium between myocardial oxygen supply and myocardial demand must be restored to relieve the symptom.[12]

ETIOLOGY

   The cause of the chest pain has not been clearly established. One theory suggests that when there is an inadequate myocardial oxygen supply, cell metabolism changes from aerobic to anaerobic. During anaerobic metabolism, lactic acid and other acids are produced as by-products; these by-products may irritate myocardial neural receptors.[12] Various diseases may decrease the coronary artery blood supply:[12]

1. Coronary atherosclerosis

2. Coronary ostia stenosis

3. Anemia

4. Tachyarrhythmias

   Disease states or alterations which increase myocardial oxygen consumption include:[12]

1. Tachyarrhythmias

2. Hyperthyroidism

3. Aortic valve stenosis

4. Aortic regurgitation

Variant angina or Printzmetal angina is thought to be caused by complete occlusion of a coronary artery by arterial spasm that temporarily restricts blood flow to the heart. [5, 6] Several investigators feel that resting angina in the absence of atherosclerosis is caused by coronary artery spasms and not by an increased demand by the heart. [6]

Certain drugs have been documented to induce anginal pain by rapidly lowering blood pressure, shifting blood away from the myocardium, or by causing direct cardiotoxicity. These drugs include:

Diazoxide (IV)	Indomethacin
Hyperstat	Indocin
	Insulin
Dipyridamole (IV)	Methysergide maleate
Persantine	Sansert
Dobutamine HCl	Prazosin HCl
Dobutrex	Minipress
Dopamine	Propranolol HCl
Intropin	Inderal
5-Fluorouracil (5-FU)	Thyroid hormones
Adrucil, Efudex,	
Fluoroplex	Tolazoline HCl
	Priscoline, Vasodil
Hydralazine HCL	
Apresoline, Dralzine,	
Lopress	

ASSESSMENT SPECIFIC TO THE ALTERATION

Subjective Data (Symptoms)

During historical data collection, the client should be carefully questioned regarding the pain or discomfort which he has been experiencing. Assessment of the pain includes:

1. Bodily location   5. Setting

2. Quality   6. Aggravating factors

3. Chronology   7. Alleviating factors

4. Quantity   8. Associated symptoms

Bodily Location

The origin of the pain is in the anterior midchest or sub-sternal area. [12, 22] It is not uncommon for the pain to originate in the epigastrium, neck, jaw, shoulders, elbows, or arms. [22] The chest pain may radiate to the neck or down the left (sometimes the right) arm. [22]

Quality of the Pain

The client may describe the pain as constricting, squeezing, heaviness, tightness, pressure, indigestion, cramping, burning, sharp, aching, or indescribable. [12, 22]

Chronology

Usually the pain or discomfort associated with angina pectoris lasts for a brief period of approximately 20 minutes or less. [22] Some clients have stated that the discomfort they have experienced has lasted for longer periods up to an hour or more. [22]

Quality

The severity of the discomfort varies from client to client. Some clients have described it as a vague discomfort, while others complain of intense, immobilizing pain. [22] The pain usually is eased if the client ceases his activities and relaxes. [22] The frequency of the episodes of angina pectoris should be ascertained. The client should be asked how many nitroglycerin tablets he uses per day or week and if the chest discomfort has limited his ability to work or engage in recreational activities. [22]

Setting

It is important to discover what activities cause the client to experience chest discomfort and where he is when the discomfort usually occurs. Common activities or times which may favor the orgin of angina pectoris include:

Shaving	Sexual intercourse
Combing hair	Tension at work
Walking in cold weather	Ingesting heavy meals
Running	Attending an exciting sports event
Climbing	Arguing with someone [22]

If the event can be identified and it cannot be avoided or altered, prophylactic use of nitroglycerin may be helpful in avoiding discomfort. [22]

Aggravating or Alleviating Factors

Stress plays a significant role in the initiation of angina pectoris. The stressors must be identified and eliminated or at least controlled. Stressors include:

Exertion	Excitement
Anger	Nightmares
Fear	Exposure to cold
Pain	Heavy meals
Tension	Isometric exertion (i. e., shoveling snow, lifting heavy objects) [22]

In angina decubitus, the client experiences pain while resting in a chair or sleeping. [22] The discomfort of angina usually can be relieved or lessened by physical and emotional rest and nitroglycerin use. [22] The action of nitroglycerin is rapid, and discomfort usually is relieved immediately or within about 3 minutes. [22] Nitroglycerin may not be effective for all clients with angina pectoris, and it has been known to alleviate chest pain other than that caused by angina pectoris.

Associated Symptoms

Other symptoms besides pain may occur in angina pectoris such as palpitations, dizziness, and nausea. Clients experiencing "unstable angina" may state that the pain occurs in a pattern of increasing frequency, increasing provocation, and/or with increasing severity. [10]

Objective Data (Signs)

During an episode of acute ischemia, physical findings may include: transient tachycardia, hypertension, evidence of left ventricular dysfunction(i. e., precordial bulge, S4 or S3 gallop rhythm, paradoxical splitting of the second heart sound, a mitral regurgitation murmur or bibasilar pulmonary rales, rise in the pulmonary artery end-diastolic and pulmonary capillary wedge pressures).[10, 21]

Blood Pressure

During a spontaneous or induced anginal attack, there may be a significant elevation in the systolic and diastolic blood pressure.[14] If the blood pressure falls with the onset of ischemia, it is an indication that the left ventricle may be so severely compromised that cardiac output is greatly decreased.[10]

Electrocardiogram

The resting ECG may be normal in 25% of the clients.[14] ECG changes which indicate ischemia during anginal pain include:[10]

1. Changes in leads II, III, and aV_F (inferior leads) reflect right coronary artery disease

2. Changes in V_2 through V_5 (anterior leads) reflect left anterior descending artery disease

3. Changes in leads I, aV_L, and V_6 (lateral leads) reflect circumflex artery disease

These associations between leads and the three main arteries would not hold true if the client has variations in the normal distribution of arteries.[10] Other ECG changes often associated with angina pectoris include:

1. Peaked T wave

2. Flattened T wave

3. T wave inversion

4. ST depression with or without T wave inversion

5. ST elevation seen in Printzmetal angina [10]

Diagnostic Examinations

Laboratory tests should be done to detect anemia, hypercholesterolemia, hypertriglyceridemia, diabetes mellitus, hypoglycemia, hyperthyroidism, and syphilis.[14] A serologic test for syphilis (STS) and chest x-ray should be done routinely. Selective cineangiocardiography and exercise tests may be performed when the diagnosis is in doubt. Holter monitoring is indicated if the client is suspected of having transient rhythm or conduction disturbances during regular activities.[23] In this way, the cardiac rhythm is recorded continuously on a 12 to 24 hour cassette tape. The client keeps a record of palpitations or unusual events; this is later compared to the ECG record. Other common diseases which cause chest pain should be ruled out (i. e., peptic ulcer, chronic cholecystitis, hiatus hernia, cervical or thoracic spine disease, etc.).

CLIENT CARE GOALS

1. Equilibrium between myocardial oxygen supply and demand must be restored.

2. Pain/discomfort must be relieved.

3. Future anginal attacks will be prevented or at least decreased in frequency.

4. Stressors must be identified and eliminated or controlled.

INTERVENTIONS

Whenever possible, the underlying cause (i. e., thyrotoxicosis, aortic valvular disease, anemia, or tachyarrhythmias) should be removed.[12] If the etiology is atherosclerosis, this approach is not feasible. Client education is extremely important. Anginal attacks may be prevented if the client is taught:

1. To use moderation in all aspects of his life

2. To participate in daily activities that do not cause chest discomfort, dyspnea, and extreme fatigue

3. Overeating should be avoided

4. Physical activity should be postponed until approximately 1 hour after meals

5. Body weight should be slightly below normal

6. Known stressful situations should be avoided

7. Smoking should be eliminated

8. Cold weather should be avoided if possible or the client should dress appropriately in warm clothing

9. Carrying or lifting heavy objects should be avoided[4]

DRUG THERAPY

If the above conservative interventions are not effective, drug therapy may be initiated. The two most common types of antianginal agents are the nitrates and beta-blockers.[9] The client on drug therapy must be taught the drug's actions, side effects, dosage, mode of administration, and storage precautions. Drug therapy usually consists of the following:

Nitroglycerin

There is some disagreement in the literature as to whether or not nitroglycerin dilates the coronary arteries in the presence of coronary artery disease.[12] It appears that the primary mechanism of action in relieving anginal pain results from relaxation of the smooth muscle of the vascular system, which in turn lowers the arterial systolic pressure.[12] Because the left ventricle then pumps against a lower systolic pressure, myocardial oxygen consumption is reduced.[12] Other effects due to relaxation of smooth muscle include decreased venous tone, cardiac output, and pulmonary artery pressure.[12] There may be a compensatory increase in heart rate in response to the decreased blood pressure, but this usually is not significant.[12]

The sublingual nitroglycerin dosage varies between 0.3 mg and 0.6 mg. The onset of action is rapid, usually 2 to 3 minutes and relief may last for 10 to 30 minutes.[12] If the pain is not relieved within 5 minutes after the initial dose and rest, the client may be instructed to repeat the dose. However, no more than three tablets at 5 minute intervals should be taken. The client should be cautioned to avoid standing while taking the nitroglycerin because of the decrease in blood pressure that occurs. If pain persists, the client should call his physician. Side effects include: headache, dizziness, flushing of skin, and occasionally syncope.[12] The tablets should be stored in their original brown container with the top tightly closed. Light and moisture decrease the drug's potency. Cotton should not be placed in the container, since it absorbs nitroglycerin.[12] The

nitroglycerin supply should be renewed every 3 months to ensure potency. [4] Tablets that are potent produce a burning sensation under the tongue. [12] Sublingual nitroglycerin may be
used prophylactically to prevent anginal pain, when exercise or
emotionally stressful situations are anticipated. [4, 12]

The action of nitroglycerin ointment (2%) is the same as
sublingual nitroglycerin, but the duration of action is longer.
The dosage is individually determined for each client and is
dependent on the baseline heart rate and blood pressure values.
The ointment should not be rubbed in because this would increase the rate of absorption and decrease the duration of action. [12] Applications may be repeated every 6 hours. The ointment should be stored away from heat and with the cap firmly
replaced.

Sublingual long-acting isosorbide dinitrate preparations
(Isordil, Sorbitrate) produce hemodynamic changes similar to
those of nitroglycerin: decreased arterial systolic pressure,
decreased pulmonary artery pressure, and decreased cardiac
output. [12] Initial dosage is 2.5 mg every 3 to 4 hours. Side
effects are similar to nitroglycerin and may decrease with a
reduced dosage. [12]

Propranolol (Inderal)

Propranolol is sometimes used for clients experiencing
incapacitating episodes of angina pectoris. Propranolol blocks
sympathetic nerve stimulation; it decreases the heart rate,
atrioventricular conduction, and myocardial tension resulting
in a reduction in myocardial oxygen consumption. [12] Many
clients experience a fewer number of anginal attacks and an increase in exercise tolerance. [12] Initial oral dosage is 10 mg
every 6 hours. The dosage can be increased gradually every
2 or 3 days until the desired effect is obtained. Dosage should
be reduced gradually before the drug is discontinued; several
clients have suffered angina and myocardial infarction several
days after the abrupt withdrawal of propranolol. [12, 16] Side
effects include:

Nausea	Weakness
Vomiting	Fatigue
Diarrhea	Skin rash
Lightheadedness	Paresthesia of the hands

Constipation   Sore throat

Lassitude   Visual disturbances[8]

Drug fever

Propranolol is contraindicated if the client experiences
bronchial asthma, allergic rhinitis, sinus bradycardia, heart
block, cardiogenic shock, right ventricular failure secondary
to pulmonary hypertension, or congestive heart failure.[8] It
is contraindicated also in clients receiving heart-depressing
anesthetics. The drug should be used with caution in clients
who have diabetes mellitus; it can cause hypoglycemia and mask
the usual side effects of hypoglycemia.[12]

(See the Appendix for a review of antianginal agents in tab-
ular form.)

Complications

Diabetes mellitus, hypertension, congestive heart failure,
myocardial infarction, and arrhythmias shorten life expectancy.
Sudden death is also a possibility.[23]

REVIEW QUESTIONS

1. Describe angina pectoris.

2. Discuss "anaerobic metabolism" in relation to angina
pectoris.

3. List at least three disease states which increase myocardial oxygen consumption.

4. Define the following:

Unstable angina

Printzmetal angina

Angina decubitus

5. Describe the quality of pain frequently present when the
client is experiencing angina pectoris.

6. List possible stressors which may precipitate or aggravate anginal pain.

7. Name nine preventative steps that should be taught to the client to decrease or eliminate episodes of angina.

8. How rapid is the onset of action of sublingual nitroglycerin?

9. List four common side effects of nitroglycerin.

10. How often should the client's supply of nitroglycerin be replaced?

11. Should nitroglycerin ointment be rubbed into the skin? Explain your answer.

12. Describe the mode of action of propranolol (Inderal).

13. In what conditions is propranolol contraindicated?

14. List possible complications of angina pectoris.

REFERENCES

1. Allendorf, E. and Keegan, M. H.: Teaching Patients About Nitroglycerin. Am J Nurs 75 (July 1975): 1168.

2. Benedict, C. and Robertson, D.: Be Alert For Ergot-Induced Angina. Nurs Drug Alert 3 (December 1979): 137.

3. Boedeker, E. and Dauber, J.: Manual of Medical Therapeutics. 21st Ed., Boston: Little, Brown, and Co., 1974, p. 85.

4. Brunner, L. et al.: Textbook of Medical-Surgical Nursing. 2nd Ed., Philadelphia: J.B. Lippincott Co., 1970, pp. 371-373, 1975, 1980.

5. Carleton, R. and Johnson, A.: Coronary Arterial Spasm. Mod Conc Cardiovasc Dis 43 (May 1974): 87-91.

6. Marx, J. L.: Coronary Artery Spasms and Heart Disease. Science 208 (June 6, 1980): 1127-1130.

7. Cromwell, V. et al.: Understanding the Needs of Your Coronary Bypass Patient. Nursing 80 (March 1980): 34-45.

8. Falconer, M. et al.: The Drug-The Nurse-The Patient. 6th Ed, Philadelphia: W.B. Saunders Co., 1978, p. 296.

9. Fuller, E.: The Effect of Antianginal Drugs on Myocardial Oxygen Consumption. Am J Nurs 80 (February 1980): 250-254.

10. Gronim, S.: Helping the Client With Unstable Angina. Am J Nurs 78 (October 1978): 1677-1680.

11. Jenkins, J. W.: Primary Emergency Care For Victims of Cardiovascular Disorders. Emerg Med Tech 4 (March 1980): 55-61.

12. Kise, M.: Drug Therapy in the Treatment of Angina Pectoris. Nurs Clin N Am 11 (June 1976): 309-318.

13. Klegfield, P.: Coronary Artery Spasm: New Life For An Old Theory. Emerg Med 12 (April 30, 1980): 56-59.

14. Krupp, M. A. and Chatton, M. J.: Current Medical Diagnosis and Treatment. Los Altos, Calif.: Lange Medical Publications, 1976, pp. 187-192.

15. Likoff, W. et al.: Evaluation of Coronary Vasodilatation by Coronary Angiography. Am J Cardiol 13 (1974): 7.

16. Lipman, A.: Which Drugs May Induce Angina Pectoris? Mod Med (April 15-30, 1980): 113-114.

17. Mikolich, J. R.: Relief of Refractory Angina with Continuous Intravenous Infusion of Nitroglycerin. Chest 77 (March 1980): 375-379.

18. Miller, B. and Keane, C.: Encyclopedia and Dictionary of Medicine, Nursing and Allied Health. 2nd Ed., Philadelphia: W. B. Saunders Co., 1978.

19. Park, J. O. et al.: The Effect of Nitroglycerin on Coronary Artery Blood Flow and the Hemodynamic Response To Exercise In Coronary Artery Disease. Am J Cardiol 27 (1971): 59.

20. Pathy, M.: Propranolol-Caused Chest Pain Mimics A Heart Attack. Nurs Drug Alert 3 (December 1979): 139.

21. Rogers, W.: Current Concepts in Evaluation of Coronary Artery Disease. Hosp Med 16 (March 1980): 10-21.

22. Silverman, M. E.: Examination of the Heart. Part 1: The Clinical History. American Heart Association, Inc., 1975, pp. 11-15.

23. Sokolow, M.: Heart and Great Vessels. In Krupp, M. A. and Chatton, M.J.: Current Medical Diagnosis and Treatment. Los Altos, Calif.: Lange Medical Publications, 1976, pp. 187-193.

24. Dietz, H. L. (ed.): Symposium on Cardiac Care. Nurs Clin N Am 13 (September 1978): 387-554.

25. White, P. D.: The Historical Background of Angina Pectoris. Mod Conc Cardiovasc Dis 43 (September 1974): 109-112.

CHAPTER 9

AORTIC COARCTATION

LEARNING OBJECTIVES

Study of this chapter will enable the reader to:

1. Distinguish between preductal and postductal coarctation

2. Describe physical findings in relation to blood pressure, pulses, and murmurs in the adult client with aortic coarctation

3. Employ specific physical assessment skills to detect congenital abnormalities in the newborn, older child, and the adult client

4. Formulate a nursing care plan to promote physical and emotional rest in the client

5. Describe possible postsurgical complications

6. Describe the complications that may occur in the untreated client

DESCRIPTION

Coarctation of the aorta is characterized by deformity of the tunica media of the aorta, causing narrowing of the lumen of the vessel. [6] It occurs in one out of every 2000 people in the general population. [3] Coarctation of the aorta exists in two forms:

1. Preductal coarctation characterized by constriction of the aorta before the entrance of the ductus arteriosus.

2. Postductal coarctation (adult type) is the more common of the two types and is characterized by constriction of the aorta directly beyond the ductus arteriosus. [3, 4] In

this type of coarctation, a collateral circulation develops and bypasses the constriction to supply oxygenated blood to the lower extremities.

Frequently, other cardiac defects are seen in preductal coarctation. [4] Coarctation of the aorta is responsible for an increased left ventricular pressure and increased cardiac work load; it is classified as an "acyanotic" congenital heart abnormality.

ETIOLOGY

The cause of this congenital birth defect is unknown. [3]

ASSESSMENT SPECIFIC TO THE ALTERATION

Historical Data (Subjective Data)

Coarctation of the aorta is usually asymptomatic in childhood; growth and development may be normal. Later in life, symptoms may consist of: occasional fatigue, nosebleeds, leg cramps, headache, chest pain, and cold feet. [3]

Objective Data (Signs)

Physical examination reveals:

1. An absence of femoral pulses, but good carotid and radial pulses (this is usually a sign of coarctation of the aorta in an infant)

2. Signs of congestive failure may occur when the baby is 10 to 15 days old

3. A hypoglycemic infant due to the decreased supply of blood to the liver. [7]

Signs in the adult include:

Bounding pulses in the upper extremities.

Absent or greatly reduced femoral pulses.

Hypertension in the upper extremities.

Diminished blood pressure in the lower extremities.

Other symptoms secondary to hypertension.

Systolic murmur along the left sternal border over the base of the heart.

A high frequency murmur in the interscapular area of the back.

Pulsations arising from enlarged vessels may be visible over the interscapular area of the back in older clients.

A chest x-ray may reveal cardiomegaly in preductal coarctation or an enlarged left ventricle, dilated ascending aorta, and at times an enlarged left atrium in postductal coarctation.

Rib notching is a common finding in clients over 8 years of age. (See Figure 13 for coarctation of the aorta with rib notching).

The electrocardiogram may be normal or may reveal left ventricular hypertrophy with systolic overload.[2,3,4] A right ventricular hypertrophic pattern may be observed in infants.[4]

Diagnostic techniques include: an aortogram (procedure of choice for infants) which pinpoints the site and size of the coarctation and any associated defects; angiography and cardiac catheterization are often done.

CLIENT CARE GOALS

1. Early recognition of the congenital defect

2. Prevention of physical and emotional fatigue

3. Prevention of infections and other complications preoperatively and postoperatively

4. Maintain adequate fluid and nutritional intake

5. Correction of defect whenever possible

6. Provide regular medical follow-up to prevent future complications

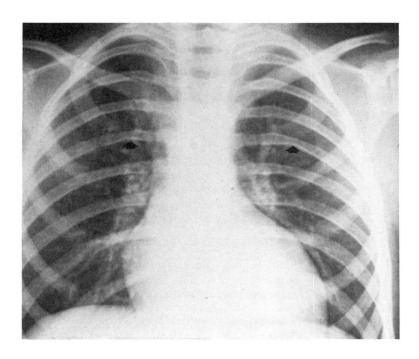

Figure 13. Coarctation of the aorta associated with rib notching. (Reprinted with permission from Anthony, C. et al. : Pediatric Cardiology — Medical Outline Series. Garden City, NY: Medical Examination Publishing Co. , Inc. , 1979, p. 128.)

INTERVENTIONS

Nursery nurses play an important role in the detection of congenital defects by routinely performing a nursing assessment of the newborn (i. e. , color, respirations, heart rate, blood pressure, presence of pulses, murmurs, ability to feed well, etc.). [7] The best time for surgical intervention is between the ages of 8 and 16 years. [3] When surgery is indicated, the coarcted area is resected with a direct anastamosis. The nurse will probably be responsible for teaching the parents how to care for their baby at home. Parent education should include an explanation of:

The type of problem their baby has

Symptoms that should be brought to the physician's attention and where to go for help if the physician is unavailable

How to count the pulse

How to administer prescribed drugs

Signs of drug toxicity

How to take the baby's temperature

How to feed the baby

How to position the baby for ease in breathing [7]

The nurse caring for the older child with a cardiac defect must try to direct the child's activity to avoid additional strain on the heart. Nursing procedures are scheduled so that the client can rest at intervals. All procedures should be explained in understandable terms and demonstrated whenever possible. It is important that the nurse:

1. Allow the child to vent his feelings

2. Provide an unhurried environment

3. Encourage the child to eat a nutritious diet and consume adequate fluids

4. Avoid exposing the child to any type of infection [4]

Preoperative Care

Immediate preoperative preparation includes:

1. Psychological preparation

2. Morning Care

3. Vital Signs

4. Adequate hydration as prescribed

5. Preoperative medication

6. Offering the bedpan before sending the child to surgery[4]

Postoperative Care

Postoperative care would be similar to that for any client following cardiac surgery (i.e., vital signs, maintaining a patent airway, oxygen therapy, intake and output, closed-chest drainage, observation for signs of hemorrhage and other complications).[3,4] A discharge conference should be planned so that the parents know:

1. What activity limits, if any, have been set by the physician

2. How to provide an adequate diet

3. The importance of dental care to prevent decay and infection

4. That the child most likely will be able to attend a regular school [4]

Most surgical corrections are recommended before adult life. Clients requiring correction of the defect in adult life are prepared preoperatively and postoperatively in a manner similar to that for any adult undergoing open-chest surgery. Although it has been stated that the condition should be treated surgically, the older, fairly asymptomatic person with a severely calcified aorta is an exception. In this case, the surgical risk outweighs the benefits.[3] The blood pressure becomes normal in about one-third of the adult clients immediately following surgery; another one-third of the clients becomes normotensive during the first week after surgery.[3] In some clients, it takes much longer before the blood pressure becomes normal and in some, it never does.[3,5] Close postoperative follow-up is mandatory to evaluate the effects of residual cardiovascular anomalies and hypertension.[5] Possible postoperative complications include: bleeding from the suture line or from a divided collateral vessel, thoracic duct damage, abdominal pain 5 to 7 days postoperatively, and weakness or paralysis of the legs (rare).[3]

COMPLICATIONS

If untreated, many clients die in early adult life from complications such as: cerebral hemorrhage, rupture of the aorta, bacterial endocarditis, or congestive heart failure.[2, 3, 4]

Adults who have had a coarctation repaired in infancy, may have a recurrent coarctation or myocardial infarction.[3]

REVIEW QUESTIONS

1. Define the following:

   Coarctation of the aorta

   Preductal coarctation

   Postductal coarctation

2. Is coarctation of the aorta classified as a cyanotic or acyanotic congenital heart abnormality?

3. Describe the physical findings in relation to femoral, carotid, and radial pulses in the client with coarctation of the aorta.

4. List the objective signs of coarctation of the aorta in the adult.

5. Is surgical intervention the intervention of choice?

6. Describe the immediate preoperative preparation of the older child with a coarctation of the aorta.

7. What items should the nurse include in a discharge conference with the child's parents?

8. What complications are possible if the condition is left untreated?

9. Name four possible postsurgical complications.

REFERENCES

1. Anthony, C. et al.: Pediatric Cardiology. Garden City, NY: Medical Examination Publishing Co., Inc., 1979, pp. 288-298.

2. Brunner, L. and Suddarth, D.: The Lippincott Manual of Nursing Practice. 2nd Ed., Philadelphia: J.B. Lippincott Co., 1978, pp. 1548-1549.

3. Comer, T.: Coarctation of the Aorta: Really Not So Rare. Consultant (April 1980): 158-161.

4. Hodgson, L.M. (ed.): Congenital Heart Abnormalities. Number 7. Columbus, Ohio: Ross Laboratories, 1972, pp. 32-35.

5. Kaplan, S.: Long-Term Results After Surgical Treatment of Congenital Heart Disease. Mod Conc Cardiovasc Dis 46 (January 1977): 3.

6. Miller, B. and Keane, C.: Encyclopedia and Dictionary of Medicine, Nursing and Allied Health. 2nd Ed. Philadelphia: W.B. Saunders Co., 1978, p. 227.

7. Moore, M. L.: Realities in Childbearing. Philadelphia: W.B. Saunders Co., 1978, p. 583.

CHAPTER 10

ARTERIOSCLEROSIS — ATHEROSCLEROSIS

LEARNING OBJECTIVES

Study of this chapter will enable the reader to:

1. Define the three main types of arteriosclerosis

2. Identify risk factors that predispose an individual to arteriosclerosis

3. Describe five of the early symptoms of arteriosclerosis

4. State the physical signs that may be observed in a client experiencing peripheral arterial disease

5. List several foods that are rich in cholesterol and saturated fats

6. Describe the mode of action and side effects of two antilipemic agents

7. Explain the specific interventions that should be implemented by the client experiencing peripheral arterial disease

8. Prepare the client to assume responsibility for his/her own physical care at home

9. Evaluate the effectiveness of the client's educational program within the health care facility

DESCRIPTION

Arteriosclerosis is a general term used to describe an arterial disease characterized by thickening and loss of the elasticity of the arterial walls. Lay people commonly refer to this alteration as "hardening of the arteries."

There are three main types or forms of arteriosclerosis:

1. Atherosclerosis is the most common type of arteriosclerosis in which plaques of fatty deposits (atheromas)
form in the inner layer (intima) of the arteries (it
chiefly affects the aorta, coronary, cerebral, and
lower extremity arteries); this alteration results in an
obstruction to the flow of blood.

2. Monckeberg arteriosclerosis (medial arteriosclerosis)
involves the middle layer (medial coat) of the arteries;
there is destruction of the muscle and elastic fibers of
the medial coat and calcium deposits.

3. Arteriolar sclerosis (arteriolosclerosis) affects the
arterioles.[8]

Atherosclerosis is more common in men than in women;
the rate increases in women after the menopause.[2] It appears
that estrogen protects the female.[6] Hudak et al. state that
approximately 95% of all cases of myocardial damage are due
to intrinsic disease of the coronary vessels as a result of
arteriosclerotic changes in the vessel walls.[6]

ETIOLOGY

It is generally thought that a combination of factors contribute to the disease process. Heredity may play a part in
predisposing an individual to arteriosclerosis.[1, 3, 8]

Risk factors include:

Age

Sex (death rate in white
males 34 to 44 years of
age is six times greater
than in females)

Emotional tension

Elevated serum lipids

Hypertension

Diabetes mellitus

Hypothyroidism

Gout (uric acid levels
6.9 mg/100 ml and above)

Cigarette smoking

Obesity

Physical inactivity

Some authorities report that
the softer the drinking water,
the higher the mortality from
cardiovascular conditions.[2, 3,6]

Hudak et al. state that any situation eliciting a sympathetic or adrenal stress response may contribute to the establishment of the conditions prerequisite for the development of
atherosclerotic changes in the coronary circulation. [6]

ASSESSMENT SPECIFIC TO THE ALTERATION

Subjective Data

The nurse collecting the client's historical data should be
very careful to obtain information regarding the presence of
risk factors and the client's dietary habits. The client's symptoms will depend upon which of the arteries are affected by arteriosclerosis. Early symptoms may include: coldness or
numbness in the feet, dizziness, dyspnea, headache, and fatigue. [8]

If the legs are affected, the client may complain of leg
cramps, aches, and sharp pains after mild exercise. [8] If cerebral arteries are involved, mental symptoms such as memory
loss may develop. [8] Since arteriosclerosis is the major cause
of other diseases such as angina pectoris, myocardial infarction, cerebral vascular accident, and peripheral thrombosis,
the symptoms and signs would be related to the specific disorder and are discussed under those topics.

Objective Data

The physical signs would be specific to the alteration or
disease process being experienced by the client. Signs observed
in the client experiencing peripheral arterial disease include:

1. Alterations in color and/or temperature of the affected
   extremities

2. Inadequate nutrition of the limb as evidenced by thick,
   opaque nails; shiny and atrophic skin; decreased hair
   growth; dry or fissured heels; and loss of subcutaneous
   tissue in the toes. [7, 9]

Peripheral arteries (i.e., femoral, popliteal, dorsalis
pedis, posterior tibial) should be palpated and a comparison
made between both sides of the body. Absence of palpable
pulses is one of the most reliable signs of occlusive arterial
disease. [7] The arterial wall being palpated should also be
assessed for tortuosity and calcium deposits. A systolic bruit

heard on auscultation of the major arteries may indicate atheromatous plaques. [7] Other diagnostic tests which are commonly done include oscillometry to help pinpoint the level of arterial occlusion, reactive hyperemia test (skin temperature studies), arteriography, exercise tests for intermittent claudication, and lumbar sympathetic block. [1, 7] Laboratory studies may reveal the presence of hyperlipoproteinemia.

CLIENT CARE GOALS

1. Prevention of atherosclerosis if possible by decreasing known risk factors.

2. Prevention of the progression of the disease process once it is detected.

3. Promotion of physical and emotional comfort.

4. Continued total assessment of the client to prevent complications.

INTERVENTIONS

Refer to the chapters on angina pectoris, myocardial infarction and cerebral vascular accident for specific interventions related to these alterations. Generally speaking, the focus of care should be directed at prevention of or delaying the progression of the disease process. The nurse should assist the client in the identification and reduction or elimination of risk factors (i.e., emotional tension, obesity, cigarette smoking, hypertension, diabetes mellitus, and hyperlipoproteinemia). [3]

Diet

Dietary management may be considered, since diets rich in cholesterol and saturated fats elevate serum cholesterol levels. Foods containing saturated fats should be avoided or restricted as prescribed by the physician. These foods include:

Beef	Hydrogenated shortenings
Lamb	Cream
Pork	Margarine

Veal   Butter

Whole milk   Chocolate[2]

Ice cream

Drugs

Antilipidemic drugs may be used as adjuncts to diet therapy in all types of hyperlipoproteinemia except type I.

Clofibrate (Atromid-S) is prescribed most often in a dosage of 500 mg four times daily. The mode of action is thought to be that of inhibiting the hepatic release of lipoproteins and inhibiting cholesterol biosynthesis.[2] Side effects include nausea, vomiting, diarrhea, dyspepsia, and abdominal distress.[2]

Clofibrate increases the action of coumarin anticoagulants and therefore the dosage of the anticoagulant should be lowered. Clofibrate should not be administered in the presence of hepatic disease. Malabsorption of vitamin B_{12}, iron, and electrolytes has occurred with this drug.[2]

Niacin (nicotinic acid) is a vitamin which appears to lower cholesterol and triglyceride levels by reducing the rate of synthesis of beta-lipoprotein.[2] Side effects include: intense flushing, headaches, pruritis, jaundice, and abnormal liver function tests. It is also contraindicated in the presence of liver disease. Other antilipemic agents are available.

Vasodilators and anticoagulants also may be prescribed. If this is the case, the client must be taught what he is taking, why he is taking it, what the action is, the drug's side effects, the correct dosage, and the route of administration, as well as any precautions that should be taken.

Specific Interventions

The client should:

1. Begin a program of graduated exercise to enhance collateral circulation

2. Improve dietary habits to avoid obesity

3. Take meticulous care of the feet, using warm water, drying gently, using skin lubricants, wearing clean socks/stockings daily, and properly fitted shoes

4. Never go barefoot

5. Never wear constricting garments (garters, girdles, etc.)

6. Avoid the use of heating pads and water bottles [7]

Surgery

Surgical intervention may be considered if the chronic reduction of circulation is due to narrowing of the abdominal aorta or distal arteries in the extremities and the client is severely incapacitated. [7] The diseased arterial segment may be replaced or a bypass graft done to relieve the occlusion. These surgical procedures are not without risk. Clients usually are placed in the intensive care unit and placed on a cardiac monitor following surgery. [1] Before discharge, the client should be taught proper foot care, the hazards of prolonged sitting with the hips and knees flexed, and the signs of vascular insufficiency—coldness, numbness, pain, color changes, unhealed sores, or edema. [1] The client should be instructed to contact the physician immediately should these signs occur.

COMPLICATIONS

Complications depend on the extent of the pathology and the area of involvement. Occlusion of a bypass graft is a distinct possibility.

REVIEW QUESTIONS

1. Define the following terms:

   Arteriosclerosis

   Atherosclerosis

   Mönckeberg arteriosclerosis

   Arteriolar sclerosis

2. Name at least ten risk factors which may predispose an individual to arteriosclerosis.

3. What are some of the early symptoms that may occur in arteriosclerosis?

4. Ateriosclerosis is the major cause of other diseases. Name at least four of these diseases.

5. What are some of the signs that may be observed in the client experiencing peripheral arterial disease?

6. Name at least ten foods which contain saturated fats.

7. Describe the mode of action of clofibrate (Atromid S).

8. Does clofibrate have an effect on the action of coumarin anticoagulants?

9. Name five side effects of niacin (nicotinic acid).

10. State six specific interventions which should be implemented by the client experiencing peripheral vascular disease.

REFERENCES

1. Atchison, J. and Murray, J.: Post-Vascular Surgery, When Happiness Can Be A Warm Foot. Nursing 78 (December, 1978): 36-39.

2. Beyers, M. and Dudas, S.: The Clinical Practice of Medical-Surgical Nursing. Boston: Little, Brown, and Co., 1977, pp. 342-345.

3. Brunner, L. and Duddarth, D.: The Lippincott Manual of Nursing Practice. 2nd Ed., Philadelphia: J.B. Lippincott Co., 1978, p. 434.

4. Diethrich, E.: Pre-Infarction Syndrome—Surgical Indications. Heart Lung 4 (May-June 1975): 390-396.

5. Gotto, A.: Recognition and Management of the Hyperlipoproteinemias. Heart Lung 1 (July-August 1972): 508-518

6. Hudak, C., Lohr, T., Gallo, B.: Critical Care Nursing. 2nd Ed., Philadelphia: J.B. Lippincott Co., 1977, 84-85.

7. Luckmann, J. and Sorensen, K.: Medical-Surgical Nursing: A Psychophysiologic Approach. Philadelphia: W.B. Saunders Co., 1974, pp. 814-816, 1980, 1105-1112.

8. Miller, B. and Keane, C.: Encyclopedia and Dictionary of Medicine, Nursing and Allied Health. 2nd Ed., Philadelphia: W.B. Saunders Co., 1978, pp. 69-70.

9. Murray, R. et al.: The Nursing Process in Later Maturity. Englewood Cliffs, NJ: Prentice-Hall, Inc., 1980. pp. 231-232, 456-457.

10. Weir, R. et al.: Nursing Care Study: Lower Limb Ischaemia. Nurs Times 75 (May 24, 1979): 865-868.

11. Zamorano, C. and Diethrich, E.: Surgical Correction of Coronary Arterial Disease Associated With Lesions of the Aorta and Its Major Branches. Heart Lung 4 (May-June 1975): 402-408.

CHAPTER 11

BUERGER DISEASE

LEARNING OBJECTIVES

Study of this chapter will enable the reader to:

1. Describe the pathophysiologic changes that take place in Buerger disease

2. Describe the usual symptoms of arterial insufficiency

3. List the common objective data (signs) expected in a client experiencing Buerger disease

4. Discuss noninvasive and invasive diagnostic techniques that can be employed

5. Formulate a health teaching plan aimed at preventing or delaying the progression of the disease process

6. Recommend specific foot care safety precautions to prevent infection and tissue damage

7. Discuss conservative interventions commonly employed to correct/improve the client's status

8. Evaluate planned interventions to determine their effectiveness in assisting the client

DESCRIPTION

Buerger disease is also known as "thromboangitis obliterans." It is a disease which affects the medium-sized blood vessels and is characterized by:

1. Inflammation

2. Thickening of the vascular walls

3. Occlusive thrombosis, particularly of the lower extremities [1, 7]

Both arteries and veins are destroyed and gangrene can develop. [9] The disease <u>primarily effects</u> younger males between
the ages of 20 to 45 years. [2,9] The lower extremities are usually affected first, but vascular changes may occur in the hands
and later in the entire body. [9] The onset may be gradual or sudden. [2] Acute episodes are followed by definite remissions. [4]

ETIOLOGY

The cause of Buerger disease is unknown, however smoking
aggravates the condition and may be the cause of the disease in
clients who are sensitive to inhaled smoke. [1,9] Some authors
suggest that a <u>collagen disorder</u> may be responsible for this
disease. [4]

ASSESSMENT SPECIFIC TO THE ALTERATION

Subjective Data

The symptoms are primarily those of arterial insufficiency. [4]
The predominant symptom is <u>pain</u>. [1] The client commonly complains of intermittent <u>claudication</u> in the arch of the foot, palm
of the hand, or calf of the leg which is relieved by rest. [1,2,4]
As the disease progresses, "rest pain" is common and often
interferes with the client's ability to sleep and eat. Other common symptoms include: numbness, diminished sensation, prick-
ing and burning sensations, and coldness of the extremities. [1,2,4]

Objective Data

Signs include:

1. When the extremity is elevated above heart level,
   <u>pallor</u> is observed.

2. <u>Rubor</u> occurs when the extremity is placed in a dependent position.

3. <u>Trophic changes</u> may be apparent on inspection of the
   extremity: poor nail growth with thickening of the
   nails, loss of hair, and dry scaly skin.

4. <u>Ischemic ulceration</u> often follows trauma to the affected
   extremity.

5. Palpation reveals diminished or absent peripheral pulses (e.g., dorsalis pedis, posterior tibial, ulnar, and radial).

6. Segments of the veins may be tender, and the skin cold to touch.[2, 3, 4, 11]

Vascular changes are often asymmetric. Auscultation of the major arteries may reveal a "bruit" due to turbulent blood flow through partially occluded blood vessels.[11]

Diagnostic Examinations

Noninvasive aids include the use of:

An oscillometer to measure volume changes (this is accomplished by placing a sphygmomanometer cuff around the knee and ankle; a client with significant ischemia rarely has more than two units of oscillometric deflection at the ankle

A Doppler sensor device to detect blood flow in smaller arteries

The Allen test which is sometimes performed to demonstrate arterial occlusion of the radial or ulnar arteries[2, 3, 5]

Invasive techniques include the use of angiography which has the advantage of demonstrating the arterial supply to the lower extremities from the level of the renal arteries to the feet.[3] The following information may be obtained through the use of angiography.

1. The location of the occlusion

2. The length of the occlusion

3. The condition of the blood vessels above and below the occlusion

4. Whether a collateral blood supply exists

5. The best level for amputation, if necessary [3]

CLIENT CARE GOALS

1. Circulation in the extremities will be maintained or improved.

2. Progression of the disease process will be prevented or slowed.

3. Infection and tissue damage will be prevented

4. There will be less discomfort due to ischemia.

5. Client self-care/management will be taught and encouraged.

INTERVENTIONS

Health teaching is a priority intervention for the client experiencing Buerger disease. The client must be taught ways to maintain or improve circulation in his extremities. It is imperative that the client abstain from using tobacco since smoking increases peripheral vasoconstriction, which in turn, increases vascular resistance resulting in a reduced blood flow to the extremities.[8] The client should also avoid:

Exposure to extremely cold weather, if possible

Elevating the legs above heart level

Sitting with the legs crossed

Tight clothing

Improperly fitted shoes and hosiery [8]

Buerger-Allen exercises and progressive ambulation may be prescribed by the physician. The nurse may be responsible for teaching the client these exercises.

To accomplish the goal of preventing or delaying the progression of the disease process, the client may have to:

1. Alter his usual dietary habits and restrict him/herself to some type of fat controlled diet, which is adequate in protein, vitamin B_{12} and vitamin C to maintain tissue integrity.

2. Keep existing medical conditions (e.g., diabetes mellitus, hypertension) under control.

3. Participate in a planned exercise program. [8, 12]

The client who is being controlled on antihypertensive agents should understand that an adequate systemic arterial pressure is required in order to maintain circulation and prevent ischemic damage to the extremities. [8] Therefore, the importance of medical follow-up should be stressed. Meticulous foot care and simple safety precautions can be taught to the client, so that infection and tissue damage are avoided. Points to remember regarding foot care include:

Feet should be washed daily in tepid water with a mild soap: hot or cold temperatures should be avoided.

The feet should be patted dry gently and then lubricated with lanolin, petroleum jelly, or vegetable oil.

Lamb's wool may be placed between the toes to reduce friction and moisture.

Clean hosiery should be worn daily.

Shoes should fit properly.

Feet should be inspected daily.

Toenails should be trimmed straight across to prevent tissue injury and ingrown toenails.

If there is any sign of infection or irritation, the client should contact his physician immediately. [8]

The client should be cautioned not to walk around the house with bare feet because this increases the risk of injury to the toes and feet. Many hospitalized clients find that a bed cradle used to keep the weight of the bedclothes off the feet provides some degree of comfort.

Dr. Van der Molen of the Netherlands reports some degree of success using intra-arterial treatment in addition to the previously mentioned conservative interventions. Intra-arterial therapy involves the administration of 1% lidocaine (Xylocaine) in the femoral arteries. [12]

Surgical intervention may be necessary. A sympathectomy is of value in eliminating the vasoconstrictive manifestations of the disease. [4] The procedure is said to assist in the development of collateral circulation and it may relieve some forms of intermittent claudication and rest pain.[4] Client's experiencing Buerger disease may not require amputation, if they give up smoking and are carefully managed.

COMPLICATIONS

Complications include gangrene and amputation.

REVIEW QUESTIONS

1. Describe Buerger disease.

2. In this alteration, are the arteries or the veins affected?

3. Does smoking affect the disease process?

4. What is the predominant symptom in Buerger disease?

5. List at least five common symptoms of Buerger disease.

6. Describe the following:

   Bruit
   Oscillometer
   Doppler sensor
   Allen test

7. What information can be obtained through the use of angiography in evaluation of the lower extremities?

8. Health teaching is a priority intervention for the client experiencing Buerger disease. In what ways can the client maintain or improve circulation in his extremities?

9. List eight points to remember regarding foot care.

10. What are the two dreaded complications of Buerger disease?

REFERENCES

1. Beyers, M. and Dudas, S.: The Clinical Practice of Meddical-Surgical Nursing. Boston: Little, Brown and Co., 1977, p. 403.

2. Brunner, L. and Suddarth, D.: The Lippincott Manual of Nursing Practice. 2nd Ed., Philadelphia: J.B. Lippincott Co., 1978, pp. 436-437.

3. DeWolfe, V. G.: Assessment of the Circulation in Occlusive Arterial Disease of the Lower Extremities. Mod Conc Cardiovasc Dis 45 (April 1976): 91-95.

4. Erskine, J. M.: Blood Vessels and Lymphatics. In Krupp, M. A. and Chatton, M. J.: Current Medical Diagnosis and Treatment. Los Altos, Calif.: Lange Medical Publications, 1976, pp. 256-257.

5. Fenn, J. E.: Reconstructive Arterial Surgery for Ischemic Lower Extremities. Nurs Clin N Am 12 (March 1977): 129-142.

6. Friedman, H. H. (Ed.): Problem-Oriented Medical Diagnosis. Boston: Little, Brown and Co., 1975, p. 134.

7. Miller, B. and Keane, C.: Encyclopedia and Dictionary of Medicine, Nursing and Allied Health. 2nd Ed., Philadelphia: W. B. Saunders Co., 1978, p. 155.

8. Sexton, D.: The Patient With Peripheral Arterial Occlusive Disease. Nurs Clin N Am 12 (March 1977): 89-99.

9. Shafer, K. et al.: Medical-Surgical Nursing. 6th Ed., St. Louis: C. V. Mosby Co., 1975, p. 387.

10. Sexton, D. L. (ed.): Symposium on Patients With Peripheral Vascular Disease. Nurs Clin N Am 12 (March 1977): 87-168.

11. Taggart, E.: The Physical Assessment of the Patient With Arterial Disease. Nurs Clin N Am 12 (March 1977): 109-117.

12. Van der Molen, H. R.: Vasoactive Intra-Arterial Therapy in Peripheral Occlusive Arterial Disease. Angiology 31 (April 1980): 221-229.

CHAPTER 12

CARDIAC ARRHYTHMIAS

LEARNING OBJECTIVES

Study of this chapter will enable the reader to:

1. Define the term "cardiac arrhythmia"

2. Identify specific data that should be collected during the general nursing assessment of the client

3. Describe common arrhythmias arising in the sinus node, atria, ventricles, and AV node

4. Differentiate between lethal and nonlethal arrhythmias

5. Describe interventions appropriate for each arrhythmia

6. Review the technique of basic life support (CPR) and advanced life support

7. Classify artificial pacemakers according to their rate of pacing activity

8. Plan nursing interventions following a pacemaker insertion

9. Recognize signs of pacemaker battery depletion

10. Describe possible complications following pacemaker insertion

11. Evaluate nursing and medical interventions in relation to the client's biologic and psychologic adaptation to the alteration

12. Recommend alternative actions if the client's needs have not been met effectively

GENERAL DESCRIPTION

The term arrhythmia implies that there is a disorder or alteration of the heart beat; the alteration may include a disturbance of the heart rate, heart rhythm, or both. [4] Arrhythmias may be classified as those that occur due to:

1. A disturbance in impulse formation (i.e., impulse formation arises from a pacemaker other than the sinoatrial node (SA node)

2. A conduction disturbance (i.e., transmission of the impulse is delayed, not conducted, or blocked at the affected site)

3. Combined disorders (i.e., abnormally rapid impulse formation and inability to conduct all the impulses being formed) [4]

Arrhythmias occur in normal, healthy hearts, as well as in diseased ones.

ETIOLOGY

Specific arrhythmias can be caused by factors such as:

Exercise

Infections

Fluid and electrolyte imbalances

Cigarette smoking

Drugs

Emotional states

Coffee

Disturbances of other organ systems (i.e., disease of the central nervous system causing sympathetic and vagal stimulation of the heart, pulmonary disease, endocrine disease, anemia, or renal disease. [3, 4]

Etiology will be mentioned further under the specific arrhythmia being discussed.

ASSESSMENT SPECIFIC TO THE ALTERATION

Subjective Data

General nursing assessment should include subjective data collection which would be enhanced by determining:

1. How does the client describe his symptom?

2. How frequently does the client experience the arrhythmia and how long does it last?

3. Is there any history of congestive heart failure or other known heart disease, or noncardiac diseases such as: hyperthyroidism, drug administration, electrolyte imbalance, or pacemaker implantation? [4, 5]

Objective Data

Objective data collection involves making a determination of how well the client is tolerating the arrhythmia which is evidenced by:

1. The client's general appearance

2. Whether carotid pulsation is visible

3. Auscultation of heart sounds

4. Vital signs

5. Palpation of peripheral pulses

6. Assessment of mental status

7. Presence of chest pain or discomfort

8. Respiratory effort [4, 5]

(See the specific arrhythmia being presented for more specific presenting signs).

ARRHYTHMIAS ARISING IN THE SINUS NODE

Sinus Tachycardia (Figure 16)

Description

The heart rate may be from 100 to 180 beats per minute; the rhythm is regular.[13, 20] This arrhythmia is usually harmless, unless the client has an underlying cardiac alteration.[13]

Etiology

Sinus tachycardia can be caused by any factor or state which causes stress such as: exercise, excitement, anxiety, fever, anemia, hyperthyroidism, injected drugs (i.e., atropine, epinephrine), or congested heart failure.[4, 13, 20, 25]

Subjective Data

The client's only symptom may be a feeling that his heart is racing.[13]

Objective ECG Data

The heart rate may be from 100 to 160 (some authorities state 180) beats per minute.

The rhythm is regular.

The P wave is normal in configuration and upright in lead II.

The PR intervals are of normal duration (0.12 to 0.20 second).

Each QRS complex is preceded by a P wave.[4, 20]

Interventions

Interventions are directed toward the primary cause, which is usually noncardiac.[4] Sedatives may be ordered.[13] If the client is experiencing congestive heart failure, digitalis and diuretics may be prescribed.[20] (These drugs may be found in the Appendix in this text.)

Sinus Bradycardia (Figure 15)

Description

The heart rate is below 60 beats per minute; all impulses arise in the SA (sinoatrial) node. [4,13,20] All complexes are normal in configuration. This arrhythmia may be present in both healthy and diseased hearts.

Etiology

Sinus bradycardia commonly and normally is seen during sleep and in athletes whose hearts are enlarged because of excessive exercise. [13,20,25] Other causes of sinus bradycardia include: severe pain, myxedema, acute myocardial infarction, ingestion of certain drugs such as propranolol, digitalis, morphine, etc., and "sick sinus" syndrome. [4,13]

Objective ECG Data

The heart rate is below 60 beats per minute.

The rhythm is regular.

The P wave is normal in configuration and upright in lead II.

The PR intervals are of normal duration (0.12 to 0.20 second)

Each QRS complex is preceded by a P wave. [13,20]

Interventions

Interventions usually are not necessary unless symptoms are present. If the client exhibits signs of poor cardiac output or heart failure, atropine 0.4 mg intramuscularly or intravenously may be prescribed to block the vagal effect; isoproterenol 0.2 mg. to 1.0 mg in 250 to 500 cc of 5% glucose in water may be administered IV to increase the heart rate and/or the use of a pacemaker may be necessary if the client's condition becomes refractory to treatment. [4,13,20] (See p. 146 for a review of pacemakers.)

Complications

Stokes-Adam syndrome or congestive heart failure can occur. [4]

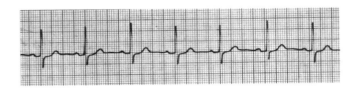

Figure 14. Normal sinus rhythm at a rate of 75 beats per minute. (Reprinted with permission from Sanderson, R. G. : The Cardiac Patient. Philadelphia: W. B. Saunders Co. , 1972.)

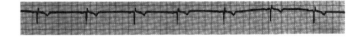

Figure 15. Sinus bradycardia at a rate of 40 beats per minute (lead V1). (Reprinted with permission from Sanderson, R. G. : The Cardiac Patient. Philadelphia: W. B. Saunders Co. , 1972)

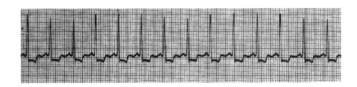

Figure 16. Sinus tachycardia at a rate of 115 beats per minute. (Reprinted with permission from Sanderson, R. G. : The Cardiac Patient. Philadelphia: W. B. Saunders Co. , 1972.)

ARRHYTHMIAS ARISING IN THE ATRIA

Premature Atrial Contractions (Figure 17)

Description

Premature atrial contractions (PACs) are common rhythm disturbances which can be seen in both healthy and diseased hearts.[4] They are of little significance unless they occur frequently; frequent PACs may precede more serious arrhythmias. PACs originate somewhere in the atrium outside of the sinus node; they occur earlier than expected in the cardiac cycle.[4, 13, 25]

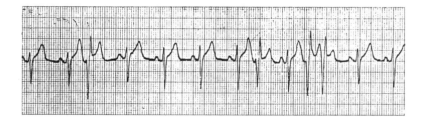

Figure 17. Beat 3 is premature and is preceded by a T wave which is deformed and more peaked than usual, due to a superimposed P wave. Note that this QRS complex is slightly aberrant. This is, therefore, an atrial premature contraction with aberrant ventricular conduction. Beat 8 is a similar premature beat and beats 10 and 11 are a pair of premature atrial contractions. The initial 0.04 second of premature beats 10 and 11 is negative and represents a Q wave. This may be evidence of myocardial infarction, or may simply represent aberrant ventricular conduction. Premature atrial beats are usually benign, but in this setting, may be a precursor to a supraventricular tachycardia or atrial fibrillation. (Reprinted with permission from Frieden, J. and Rubin, I.: ECG Case Studies. 2nd Ed., Garden City, NY: Medical Examination Publishing Co., Inc., 1974, pp. 19, 20).

Etiology

PACs may be caused by any factor causing vagal stimulation such as: heavy meals, alcohol, caffeine, or tension. Bigeminy may be found if the digitalized client has a low serum potassium.[17, 20, 25] PACs may be caused by any disease process that irritates the atrial tissues.[20]

Subjective Data

The client may state that a pause or skip in rhythm is experienced.[13]

Objective ECG Data

The P wave configuration may be abnormal.

The R to R interval of the premature beat is shorter than normal.

The PR interval may be longer or shorter than normal.

The pause following the PAC is non-compensatory.

The QRS complex is normal.[4, 13, 20]

Interventions

No treatment may be necessary; if the cause is known, it should be removed or eliminated. Mild sedation may be prescribed. Potassium replacement may be necessary, if a low potassium level is a factor.[20] Digitalis should be withheld if digitalis toxicity is suspected. Quinidine may be prescribed to suppress atrial ectopic beats.[4] Propranolol may be given if PACs occur in short runs of atrial tachycardia.[20]

Paroxysmal Atrial Tachycardia (Figure 18)

Description

Paroxysmal atrial tachycardia (PAT) is a common tachycardia which is benign in normal, healthy people; however, when it occurs in the cardiac client, a more serious arrhythmia may follow.[20] PAT is characterized by a rapid heart rate ranging from 140 to 250 beats per minute.[25] The pacemaker is in an ectopic focus of the atrium outside the sinus node.[4]

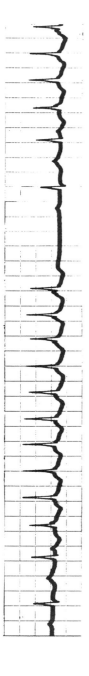

Figure 18. The first P wave is conducted with a prolonged PR interval of 0.28 second. The second P wave appears premature and is followed by a QRS after 0.28 second. The next P wave is more premature with a prolonged PR interval of 0.32 sec. The next P wave follows immediately after the third QRS and also has a prolonged PR interval. The ventricular rate becomes rapid and regular at 185/min. The P waves superimpose on various portions of the preceding QRS. After this run of tachycardia there is a long pause followed by a P wave with a prolonged PR interval. The process is then repeated. The onset of this tachycardia with a premature P wave and a prolonged PR interval is characteristic of PAT. (Reprinted with permission from Frieden, J. and Rubin, I.: ECG Case Studies 2nd Ed., Garden City, NY: Medical Examination Publishing Co., Inc., 1974, pp. 185,186.)

Etiology

The causes are similar to those causing premature atrial contractions. Rheumatic heart disease, acute myocardial infarction, or digitalis intoxication may set the stage for this arrhythmia. [13]

Subjective Data

The client may complain of dyspnea, angina pectoris, and symptoms of congestive heart failure. [13]

Objective ECG Data

The onset is sudden and frequently initiated by a premature atrial contraction.

P waves may be abnormal in contour or buried in the QRS complex.

The QRS complex is of normal configuration, but may be narrow.

The ventricular rhythm is regular; atrial rate is 160 to 250. [13, 20]

Interventions

The vagal reflex may be elicited by the Valsalva maneuver or carotid sinus pressure (performed by the physician). [13] Digitalis and diuretics may be used to prevent congestive heart failure in prolonged tachycardia. [20] Antiarrhythmic agents or countershock may be indicated in certain circumstances. [13]

Atrial Flutter (Figure 19)

Description

Atrial flutter is an arrhythmia characterized by a rapid, regular fluttering of the atrium. [4] The P waves appear to have a sawtooth pattern due to the rapid impulses arising from an ectopic focus in the atrium. [4] There is some disagreement

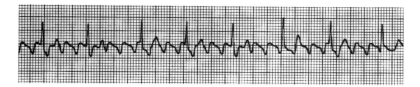

Figure 19. Atrial flutter with varying block. The atrial "flutter" waves are regular at 285 per minute. The ventricular response is irregular, the degree of block varying between 3:1 and 4:1. (Reprinted with permission from Sanderson, R. G. The Cardiac Patient. Philadelphia: W. B. Saunders Co. , 1972, p. 173.)

among cardiologists as to whether the impulse originates from multiple ectopic foci (referred to as "circus movement") or from a single ectopic focus. [13, 20] The atrial rate is very rapid between 250 and 350 impulses per minute; the ventricular rate is usually one-half of the atrial rate because the AV node is not able to accept and conduct each impulse to the ventricles. If the arrhythmia continues, further AV block develops and the ventricles respond irregularly. [13]

Etiology

The client experiencing atrial flutter usually has some underlying cardiac disease such as: coronary artery disease, cor pulmonale, or rheumatic heart disease. [13]

Objective ECG Data

The atrial rate is between 250 and 350 beats per minute.

The ventricular rate varies depending on the degree of AV block.

The ventricular rhythm is usually regular, but can be irregular depending on the conduction ratio; there may be two or more impulses for each ventricular response (2:1 ratio or 3:1 ratio).

Sawtooth flutter waves (F waves) are apparent and are uniform in width.

The QRS complex is usually normal in configuration, but narrow.[4, 13, 20]

Interventions

If the ventricular rate is rapid, digitalis is the initial drug of choice. This causes the AV node to become partially blocked, and results in a decreased pulse rate allowing more time for the heart to fill adequately before contraction.[4, 13] The atrial flutter may convert to atrial fibrillation which can be treated with quinidine.[13, 20] Countershock or atrial pacing may be indicated if the client does not tolerate the arrhythmia well and more immediate action is required.[13, 20] Caution is advised if the client is taking digitalis, because cardioversion could precipitate a fatal arrhythmia.[4]

Atrial Fibrillation (Figure 20)

Description

Atrial fibrillation is characterized by an extremely rapid and uncoordinated rate of approximately 400 to 600 impulses per minute and a grossly irregular ventricular rhythm.[4, 13, 20] The ventricles are not able to respond to every atrial impulse; only a small percentage of the atrial impulses are conducted through the ventricles.[4] The irregular ventricular rate may vary between 140 and 170 beats per minute.[13]

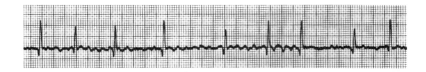

Figure 20. Atrial fibrillation with a moderate ventricular response (lead V1). Reprinted with permission from Sanderson, R. G.: The Cardiac Patient. Philadelphia: W. B. Saunders Co., 1972, p. 174.

Etiology

Transient atrial fibrillation may occur in young healthy people.[13] Permanent atrial fibrillation is associated with under-lying heart disease such as arteriosclerotic or rheumatic heart disease.[4,13]

Objective ECG Data

The atrial rate is above 400 beats per minute.

The ventricular rate is variable, 140 to 170 beats per min-ute; rhythm is completely irregular.

P waves are absent; irregular "fibrillatory" waves (f waves) are seen.

Fibrillatory waves are different in configuration because they originate from different foci in the atrium.

The PR interval is not visible.

The QRS complex may be of normal configuration.

Interventions

Cardioversion may be indicated if complications develop rapidly.[13] If the client is tolerating the arrhythmia (i.e., not hypotensive, cardiac output is sufficient, and there is no signi-ficant heart failure), digitalis may be used to increase the AV block and to increase ventricular filling time.[4,13,20] Atrial fibrillation may convert to normal sinus rhythm with the use of digitalis; quinidine may be used to maintain that rhythm.[13] Diuretics may be used if the client is in congestive heart fail-ure.[20] A temporary pacemaker has been used for selected clients who have low ventricular rates due to block.[20]

VENTRICULAR ARRHYTHMIAS

Premature Ventricular Contractions (Figure 21)

Description

Premature ventricular contractions (PVCs) occur fre-quently in normal, healthy hearts, as well as in all forms of heart disease. The PVC occurs early in the cardiac cycle and the impulse originates in the ventricles below the AV node.[4,13] PVCs occur frequently in clients who have slow heart rates. Premature ventricular contractions may be unifocal or multi-

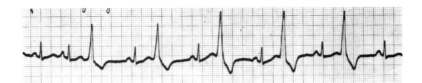

Figure 21. Ventricular premature beats in bigeminy. The PVCs
are unifocal and show fixed coupling. The second complex may be
a PAC; note that the P wave is different in configuration from
the P waves of the normal sinus beats. (Reprinted with permission from Sanderson, R. G. : The Cardiac Patient. Phil-
ladelphia: W. B. Saunders Co., 1972, p. 169.)

focal in origin. A bigeminal rhythm is present if the PVCs
occur after each sinus beat (see Figure 21); trigeminy is present if the PVCs occur after two consecutive sinus beats. 13

Etiology

PVCs may be secondary to excessive smoking, ingestion
of coffee or alcohol. 4 PVCs are especially common in clients
experiencing myocardial infarction, hypokalemia, or digitalis
intoxication. 13

Subjective Data

Some clients may be asymptomatic; others experience ventricular contractions as a thumping or skipping sensation. 13

Objective ECG Data

P waves are absent before the PVC.

The QRS complex is wide, bizarre, and distorted; it usually deflects in the opposite direction of the client's normal QRS complex.

The T wave of the PVC deflects in the opposite direction to the QRS complex.

A compensatory pause follows the premature beat. [2, 13, 20]

Interventions

If the premature ventricular contractions are infrequent and asymptomatic, no treatment is required. Multiple PVCs or PVCs falling on the peak of the T wave are treated with anti-arrhythmic agents (i. e., lidocaine, procainamide, quinidine, or propranolol.)[13] If the serum potassium is low, potassium supplement is prescribed. If digitalis toxicity is suspected, digitalis may be withheld.[13] Oxygen is administered if hypoxia is a factor.[20]

Complications

Frequent PVCs or PVCs that approach the peak of the T wave may precede or precipitate the more serious arrhythmias: ventricular tachycardia or ventricular fibrillation.[13]

Ventricular Tachycardia (Figure 22)

Description

Ventricular tachycardia is characterized by three or more consecutive, premature contractions originating from an ectopic focus below the AV node in the ventricles.[4, 25] A series of rapid, regular ventricular contractions, which are dissociated from the atrial contractions, are seen.[13] This arrhythmia may be precipitated by a PVC occurring during the vulnerable period of ventricular repolarization (called the R on T phenomenon).[20] This arrhythmia leads to a reduced cardiac output, which most clients cannot tolerate for very long; it should be treated promptly.[4, 20] Ventricular tachycardia is a precursor of ventricular fibrillation.[4]

Etiology

This arrhythmia is rarely found in normal, healthy hearts. [13] It is a common complication of myocardial infarction or digitalis intoxication. [13] As mentioned previously, this arrhythmia may be triggered if a PVC occurs during the vulnerable period of ventricular repolarization.

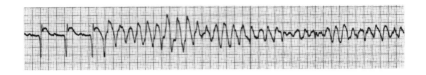

Figure 22. Ventricular tachycardia and fibrillation following a PVC which occurs during the T wave of the preceding beat. (Reprinted with permission from Sanderson, R.G.: The Cardiac Patient. Philadelphia: W.B. Saunders Co., 1972, p. 190.)

Subjective Data

The client may complain of palpitations, weakness. or angina pectoris. [13]

Objective Data

Syncope is frequently seen; hypotension and congestive heart failure may also follow due to the reduction of cardiac output. [13]

Objective ECG Data

The ventricular rate may vary from 100 to 220 beats per minute (rapid ventricular tachycardia); some authorities state the range to be from 50 (slow ventricular tachycardia) to 220 beats per minute.

R to R intervals are usually regular.

P waves are rarely seen; they may be obscured by the QRS complex.

The QRS complexes are wide and bizarre in configuration.

The T wave, when visible, is opposite in deflection to the QRS complex. [13, 20]

Interventions

A lidocaine bolus (Xylocaine) of 75 to 100 mg IV administered over a 2 minute period usually is prescribed; this may be followed by a continuous drip of lidocaine. [4] If the lidocaine is not effective, cardioversion 250 to 400 watt-sec is usually effective. [4, 13, 20] Other drugs which are sometimes prescribed to terminate the arrhythmia are: procainamide, propranolol, quinidine, diphenylhydantoin and potassium chloride. [13] If digitalis intoxication is the cause, digitalis would be stopped and potassium given. [13]

Complications

Ventricular fibrillation may follow ventricular tachycardia. If it is not terminated, death ensues. [4]

Ventricular Fibrillation (Figure 22)

Description

Ventricular fibrillation is a lethal arrhythmia characterized by rapid, irregular, ineffectual contraction of the ventricles. [4,13] Ventricular fibrillation commonly follows myocardial infarction and results in death, if it is not terminated. [4]
Since there is no cardiac output during ventricular fibrillation,
no palpable pulse is present. Ventricular fibrillation rarely
terminates spontaneously. [13]

Etiology

Ventricular fibrillation may follow myocardial infarction,
premature ventricular contractions occurring at the peak of
the preceding T wave, or toxic doses of certain drugs such as
digitalis or quinidine. [13]

Objective Data

The client loses consciousness within approximately 8 to
10 seconds after the arrhythmia begins; a seizure may occur.
A pulse is absent; pupils become dilated.

Objective ECG Data

Ventricular contractions are rapid, irregular, and ineffectual; therefore the ECG shows a wavering baseline and bizarre
waveforms.

Interventions

The best intervention is "prevention" of the arrhythmia.
Clients experiencing multiple, consecutive, or encroaching
PVCs should receive immediate treatment to prevent more serious ventricular arrhythmias. Once ventricular fibrillation
occurs, rapid defibrillation with direct current countershock
of 400 to 500 watt-sec must be performed. [13,20] If the first
shock is ineffective, another shock should be delivered within
6 seconds. [20] If the shock does not reverse the arrhythmia
immediately, cardiopulmonary resuscitation (CPR) should be
initiated. [20] Medications which should be available for the physician include: sodium bicarbonate, lidocaine, vasopressors,
epinephrine, and calcium gluconate. [20]

Complications

Death.

ATRIOVENTRICULAR BLOCKS

General Description

Atrioventricular block (AV block) refers to a conduction disturbance in which the abnormal AV node has difficulty in conducting atrial impulses into the ventricles. [4, 20] There are three types of AV block:

1. First-degree block

2. Second-degree block: Mobitz type I (also called "Wenckebach"), and Mobitz type II

3. Third-degree block (also called "complete heart block")

Etiology

Blocks may be caused by:

1. Chemicals: excessive doses of digitalis or quinidine

2. Pathologic states: myocardial infarction or degeneration of conduction tissue (as in arteriosclerotic heart disease)

3. Mechanical factors: inadvertently injuring the AV node during surgery

4. Physiologic factors: following open-heart surgery, there may be edema in the nodal region causing injury[20]

First-Degree AV Block (Figure 23)

Description

There is a delay in the conduction of the impulse from the atrium through the AV node into the ventricle. The duration of the PR interval is prolonged beyond 0.20 second. [4, 13] Once the impulse is conducted through the AV node, the ventricles respond to the impulse normally. [4, 13] This abnormality may

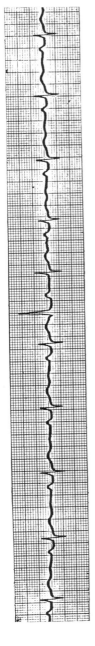

Figure 23. The rhythm is regular sinus rhythm with first-degree AV block. The PR interval is 0.24 second. Following Beat 5, there is a ventricular premature contraction which is interpolated. The ensuing PR interval is prolonged to 0.36 second. This prolongation indicates concealed retrograde conduction into the AV junction delaying the conduction of ensuing P wave. (Reprinted with permission from Frieden, J. and Rubin, I.: ECG Case Studies. 2nd Ed., Garden City, NY: Medical Examination Publishing Co., Inc. 1974, pp. 265, 266.)

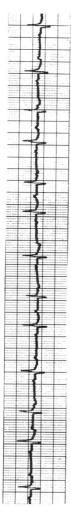

Figure 24. P waves are present at a rate of 155/min and are regular. A P wave precedes the first QRS with a PR interval of 0.16 second. The second P wave is blocked. The third P wave is conducted with a PR interval of 0.16 second. The fourth P wave is conducted with a PR interval of 0.26 second. The fifth P wave is blocked. The process is then repeated. This is second-degree heart block, Mobitz type I (Wenckebach periods), with 2:1 alternating with 3.2 AV block. The atrial mechanism is probably atrial tachycardia. (Reprinted with permission from Frieden, J. and Rubin, I.: ECG Case Studies. 2nd Ed., Garden City, NY: Medical Examination Publishing Co., Inc., 1974, pp. 167, 169.)

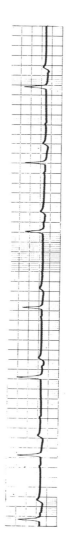

Figure 25. The PP interval is perfectly regular. The RR interval varies slightly. Each of the early QRS complexes (beats 2, 4, and 6) is preceded by a P wave with a fixed PR interval of 0.20 second. All other P waves are blocked and there are junctional escapes occurring at precisely regular RR intervals. There is a sinus rhythm with AV dissociation and occasional capture. This electrocardiogram represents a high degree of AV block (Mobitz II). Patients with this arrhythmia usually require a cardiac pacemaker. (Reprinted with permission from: Frieden, J. and Rubin, I.: ECG Case Studies. 2nd Ed. Medical Examination Publishing Co., Inc., 1974, pp. 39, 40.)

be found in all age groups and in both the healthy and diseased heart. [13]

Etiology

The PR interval may be prolonged by certain drugs such as digitalis, quinidine, and procainamide; electrolyte imbalance and ischemia of the AV node also can be a cause. [25]

Objective ECG Data

All findings are normal, except that the PR interval is prolonged beyond 0.20 second.

Interventions

Since first-degree AV block does not significantly alter cardiac output, no treatment is indicated. [13, 20]

Complications

In a severely damaged myocardium, first-degree AV block may advance to a more serious situation. [20]

Second-Degree Block; Mobitz I (Wenckebach) (Figure 24)

Description

In Mobitz I, the conduction of each impulse is progressively delayed until the sinus impulse is completely blocked and the ventricles do not respond (no QRS complex). [20] It is often said that the beat was dropped. This type of second-degree block is the more common of the two. [20]

Etiology

This type of second-degree block may be caused by inferior myocardial infarction or digitalis toxicity. [20]

Objective ECG Data

The PR interval is progressively prolonged with each beat.
The QRS complex is normal in configuration, but is progressively delayed after each P wave until one QRS complex is dropped. [13]

The dropped QRS complexes are usually cyclic so that ratios can be established. 20

Interventions

Usually no treatment is required, except to discontinue the drug if it is the cause. If the client is symptomatic, a temporary pacemaker can be inserted. 13, 20

Second-Degree Block: Mobitz II (Figure 25)

Description

Mobitz II second-degree block is characterized by a block of some sinus impulses, while some sinus impulses are conducted through the AV junction with a constant PR interval. 13 In 2:1 AV block, each QRS complex is associated with two P waves. 20 This type of block indicates a more severe type of AV-conduction impairment. 13

Etiology

Mobitz II block is seen with acute anterior myocardial infarction and suggests extensive destruction of the ventricular septum. 13, 25

Subjective Data

The client is asymptomatic unless the ventricular rate is so slow that the cardiac output is reduced. 13

Objective ECG Data

The PR interval is constant.

The QRS complex is periodically dropped because of AV block. 20

Interventions

The client should be monitored closely for progression of the block. 13 A temporary and/or permanent pacemaker may be indicated. 13, 20

Complications

This alteration may progress to third-degree heart block or ventricular standstill.

Third-Degree Block (Complete AV Block) (Figure 26)

Description

In third degree AV block, no P waves are conducted to the ventricles due to complete block at the AV junction; the atria and the ventricles beat independently of each other.[4, 20]

Etiology

Complete heart block may be congenital or acquired. Acquired cases are caused by degeneration of the conduction system due to acute myocardial infarction, myocarditis, cardiac surgery, or digitalis toxicity.[13]

Subjective Data

The client may be asymptomatic if the cardiac output is adequate (depends on the ventricular rate).

Objective Data

If the client has some form of underlying heart disease and the cardiac output becomes inadequate, heart failure may result and the client may develop Adam-Stokes seizures (i.e., ventricular tachycardia, fibrillation, or cardiac standstill resulting in syncope, hypoxic seizures, coma, or death).[13]

Objective ECG Data

The atrial rate is usually normal and regular; ventricular rate is slower and regular.

P waves are not related to QRS complexes.

The PR intervals are variable.

The QRS complex may be normal in configuration or widened depending on its area of origination.[13, 20]

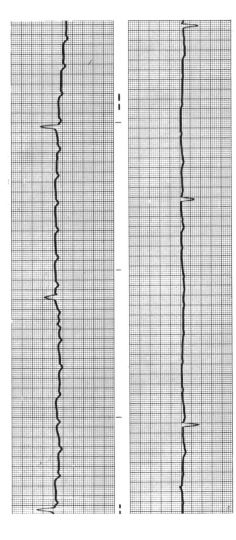

Figure 26. The atrial rate is 110 and regular. The QRS is 0.12 second. The ventricular rate is approximately 18 beats per minute and is slightly irregular. The patient has complete heart block and a very slow idioventricular pacemaker. A cardiac pacemaker should be inserted. (Reprinted with permission from: Frieden, J. and Rubin I.: ECG Case Studies. 2nd Ed. Medical Examination Publishing Co., Inc., 1974, pp. 209, 210.)

Interventions

The drug of choice is isoproterenol (Isuprel).[4, 13] A temporary or permanent pacemaker may be needed.[13] Atropine is sometimes used while the client is awaiting pacemaker insertion.[4]

Complications

The slow heart rate may predispose to PVCs and runs of ventricular tachycardia.[20]

CARDIOPULMONARY RESUSCITATION (CPR)-A REVIEW

Factors Influencing a Client's Survival

After cardiopulmonary arrest factors that influence survival include:

The time interval prior to resuscitation

The cardiorespiratory, metabolic, and neural status of the client

The client's age

Any underlying disease process

The skills and resources of the resuscitating team [18]

Basic Life Support

Basic life support involves the establishment of: an airway, breathing, and circulation.[18] These are commonly referred to as the A, B, Cs of cardiopulmonary resuscitation. One of the first steps is to determine if the victim is really unconscious by gently shaking him and trying to rouse him. If there is no response, check the victim for signs of breathing and a carotid pulse.[12] If breathing and a pulse are both absent, begin mouth-to-mouth breathing and closed-chest cardiac compression.[12] Two basic steps in giving artificial ventilation involve:

1. Opening the airway (using head tilt or jaw tilt) and checking for signs of breathing once the airway is opened.

2. Giving mouth-to-mouth ventilation (if there is one rescuer, four quick, full breaths should be given initially to the adult victim).[12]

If the victim's chest does not rise during this period, the mouth should be checked for obstructions. Airway obstructions may be removed by giving back blows, manual abdominal thrusts, and/or finger probe.[12]

After the initial four ventilations, the victim's carotid artery should be palpated for a pulse for approximately 5 seconds.[12] If the carotid pulse is absent, external cardiac compression should be initiated with the client lying on a firm surface or floor. Placement of the rescuer's hands on the sternum is important; the heel of one hand is placed on the lower half of the sternum, the other hand is placed on top and the fingers are interlocked.[12] Keeping the elbows straight, the lower sternum should be depressed $1\frac{1}{2}$ to 2 in with each cardiac compression.[12] After carrying out CPR for 1 minute, the victim's carotid artery should be palpated again for a pulse. The ratio of ventilations to cardiac compressions for one rescuer is 2:15 respectively. If two rescuers are available, the ratio is one ventilation to every five chest compressions (a compression rate of 60 per minute).[12]

Cardiopulmonary resuscitation should be continued until:

1. Circulation and ventilation are restored

2. Other medical personnel arrive to relieve you

3. You are exhausted and unable to continue resuscitation[12]

Advanced Life Support

Advanced life support consists of basic life support, using adjunctive equipment and special techniques such as:

Oxygen

Endotracheal intubation

Occasionally open-chest internal cardiac compression

Cardiac monitoring

Defibrillation

Establishing and maintaining an intravenous infusion
lifeline

Drugs and definitive therapy

Stabilization of the client's condition [19]

Drug Therapy

Essential drugs which are administered intravenously
include: sodium bicarbonate, atropine sulfate, morphine
sulfate, epinephrine, lidocaine, calcium chloride, and oxygen.[19]

Other useful drugs are the vasoactive drugs (e.g., levar-
terenol, metaraminol), isoproterenol, propranolol, and corticosteroids).[19] Termination of basic or advanced life support
is a medical decision. [19]

PACEMAKER REVIEW

Purpose and Insertion

Artificial cardiac pacemakers are used in some types of
cardiac problems in which the heart's own pacemaker (SA node)
is not functioning properly. Artificial pacemakers are useful in:

1. Controlling Stokes-Adams syndrome

2. Arrhythmias associated with myocardial infarction

3. Suppressing tachyarrhythmias

4. Postoperative cardiac surgery [3]

Artificial pacemakers may be used on a temporary or permanent basis. Both types may be inserted using the transvenous route. Veins frequently used are: the antebrachial,
jugular, femoral, or subclavian.[3] The electrode catheter is
inserted into one of these veins using fluoroscopy and is passed into
the vena cava, right atrium, and into the right ventricle.[3]
Other approaches may be used (e.g., transthoracic approach
via thoracotomy).[3]

Types

Cardiac pacemakers are classified according to the rate of pacing activity:

1. The asynchronous (fixed rate) type functions at a predetermined rate usually between 60 to 70 beats per minute; it is of limited value and may compete with the intrinsic rhythm of the heart.

2. The synchronous type has a sensing device in the atrium that triggers impulses to the ventricles after a predetermined interval; atrial disease or an atrial arrhythmia will interfere with its function.

3. Demand pacemakers are the most common type used; ventricular impulses are triggered only when the client's heart rate falls below the preset limits. 3, 7

Nursing Care of the Client After Pacemaker Insertion

Nursing interventions are aimed at:

1. Preventing catheter displacement

2. Preventing arrhythmias

3. Maintaining the pacemaker

4. Providing a safe electrical environment

5. Preventing complications such as infection, pulmonary and vascular bleeding, or hematoma

6. Client and family education regarding the pacemaker 3

Each physician and institution has its own specific protocols that should be followed after pacemaker insertion. Whenever pacemaker malfunction is suspected, a check should be made of the client's pulse rate, blood pressure, level of consciousness, and respiratory status; inadequate perfusion may cause cardiac arrest and require cardiopulmonary resuscitation. 10, 26 The client and family should be taught how to take a radial pulse for one full minute daily.

The client should be instructed to report:

1. Any irregularities in rhythm

2. Changes in pulse rate (decreases or increases in rate as determined by the physician)

3. Symptoms such as dizziness, faintness, edema, shortness of breath, and palpitations[3]

The client should know that some pacemakers may be affected by close proximity to gasoline engines, electric motors, or poorly shielded microwave ovens.[1] Referral to a public health nurse after discharge should be considered. Periodic medical check-ups are very important to monitor the function of both the client's heart and the integrity of the pacemaker.[3] Clients with pacemakers should be advised to carry a Medic-Alert card which includes the model and serial numbers of the generator and leads and the preset rate of the generator.[26]

Battery Depletion

Pulse generator failure because of battery depletion is variable according to the product's manufacturer; some batteries last for 2 to 4 years or longer. One method of accurate detection utilizes the telephone for transmission of the pulse generator rate.[7] When battery depletion occurs, the pulse rate may decrease by five to ten beats per minute from the rate set when the pacemaker was implanted.[26]

Complications

Artificial cardiac pacemakers may provoke fatal arrhythmias, perforate the myocardium, induce hiccups, thrombophlebitis, or infection.[15]

REVIEW QUESTIONS

1. Define the term "arrhythmia."

2. List at least eight factors which may be responsible for arrhythmias.

3. Describe the following arrhythmias (i.e., rate, rhythm, subjective data, etiology, ECG data):

   Sinus tachycardia

   Sinus bradycardia

   Premature atrial contraction

   Paroxysmal atrial tachycardia

   Premature ventricular contraction

   Ventricular tachycardia

   Ventricular fibrillation

   First-degree AV block

   Second-degree AV block

   Third-degree AV block

4. Describe the interventions and complications for each of the arrhythmias listed in question 3.

5. Name one of the first steps the nurse should take to determine if a client is really unconscious and in need of cardiopulmonary resuscitation (CPR)?

6. How many full breaths (mouth-to-mouth ventilations) should the lone rescuer give to the victim initially?

7. For how long should the client's carotid artery be palpated for the presence of a pulse?

8. Describe the placement of the hands on the client's sternum for chest compression when instituting CPR.

9. What is the ratio of ventilations to cardiac compressions for one rescuer? For two rescuers?

10. What does advanced life support consist of?

11. Who makes the decision to terminate basic or advanced life support?

12. Define the following:

    Asynchronous pacemaker

    Synchronous pacemaker

    Demand pacemaker

13. Describe the nursing care involved after the client has had a pacemaker inserted.

14. What steps should the nurse take if pacemaker malfunction is suspected?

15. What are some of the safety precautions that should be taught to the pacemaker client and his/her family?

16. Describe some of the complications which can arise when artificial pacemakers are in use.

REFERENCES

1. American Heart Association. Living With Your Pacemaker. Tex: American Heart Association, 1971, p. 17.

2. Arbeit, S., Rubin, I., Gross, H.: Differential Diagnosis of the Electrocardiogram. 2nd Ed., Philadelphia: F. A. Davis Co., 1975.

3. Beyers, M. and Dudas, S.: The Clinical Practice of Medical-Surgical Nursing. Boston: Little, Brown and Co., 1977, pp. 360-364.

4. Brunner, L. and Suddarth, D.: The Lippincott Manual of Nursing Practice. 2nd Ed., Philadelphia: J. B. Lippincott Co., 1978, pp. 343-405.

5. Chung, E.: How to Approach Cardiac Arrhythmias. Heart Lung 1 (July-August 1972): 523-534.

6. Conover, M.: Cardiac Arrhythmias. 2nd Ed., St. Louis: C. V. Mosby Co., 1978.

7. Escher, D.: Follow-Up of the Patient With an Implanted Cardiac Pacemaker. Mod Conc Cardiovasc Dis 43 (March 1974): 77-80.

8. Cohen, M. R. et al.: Giving Cardiovascular Drugs Safely. Horsham, Pa.: Intermed Communications, Inc., 1978.

9. Clausen, J. P. et al.: Giving Emergency Care Competently. Horsham, Pa.: Intermed Communications, Inc., 1978.

10. Hammond, C. E.: Protecting Patients with Temporary Transvenous Pacemakers. Nursing 78 8 (November 1978): 82-86.

11. Hammond, C.: Lethal Strips. RN 43 (January 1980): 54-58.

12. Hart, R.: What to do When You're Number 1: A Review of C. P. R. for Adults. Nursing 79 9 (February 1979): 54-59.

13. Hudak, C., Lohr, T., Gallo, B.: Critical Care Nursing. 2nd Ed., Philadelphia: J. B. Lippincott Co., 1977, pp. 143-161.

14. Littmann, D.: Examination of the Heart. Part V: The Electrocardiogram. New York: American Heart Association, Inc., 1973.

15. Marriott, H. and Gozensky, C.: Electrocardiogram Problems Created by Pacemakers. Cardiovasc Nurs 12 (January-February 1976): 1-6.

16. Menard, R.: Introduction to Arrhythmia Recognition. San Francisco, Ca.: California Heart Association, 1968.

17. Myerburg, R. J.: Electrocardiographic Analysis of Cardiac Arrhythmias. Hosp Prac (June 1980): 51-60.

18. Rogrove, H., Weil, M. H., Thompson, M., Blair, C.: Cardiopulmonary Resuscitation (CPR) in the Hospital. Cardiovasc Nurs 13 (March-April 1977): 7-12.

19. Moser, R. H. (ed.): Standards for Cardiopulmonary Resuscitation (CPR) and Emergency Cardiac Care (ECC). J Am Med Assoc 227 (Suppl February 18, 1974): 833-868.

20. Van Meter, M. and Lavine, P.: Reading EKG's Correctly. Nursing 77 Books, Jenkintown, Pa.: Intermed Communications, Inc., 1977.

21. Van Meter, M. and Lavine, P.: What Every Nurse Should Know About EKGs. Part I. Nursing 75 (April 1975): 19-27.

22. Van Meter, M. and Lavine, P.: What Every Nurse Should Know About EKGs. Part II. Nursing 75 (May 1975): 37-43.

23. Van Meter, M. and Lavine, P.: What Every Nurse Should Know About EKGs. Part III. Nursing 75 (June 1975): 19-25.

24. Van Meter, M. and Lavine, P.: What Every Nurse Should Know About EKGs. Part IV. Nursing 75 (July 1975): 31-37.

25. Vaz, D.: Recognizing Common Cardiac Arrhythmias. Am J Nurs 79 (November 1979): 1971-1975.

26. Viebrock, R. and Barth, F.: The Pacemaker Patient: How You Can Spare Him Needless Alarm. RN 43 (February 1980): 38-42, 117-118.

27. Westfall, U.: Electrical and Mechanical Events in the Cardiac Cycle. Am J Nurs 76 (February 1976): 231-235.

CHAPTER 13

CEREBRAL VASCULAR ACCIDENT

LEARNING OBJECTIVES

Study of this chapter will enable the reader to:

1. Distinguish between transient ischemic attacks (TIA), transient cerebral ischemic attack-incomplete recovery (TIA-IR), and completed stroke (CS)

2. Identify the three major causes of cerebral vascular accident (CVA)

3. Describe the nursing assessment which should be performed to determine the client's neurologic status

4. Describe nursing interventions to assist the client and family during the acute and rehabilitative phases of the alteration

5. Design a teaching plan to assist the client and family in recognizing and decreasing risk factors

6. Evaluate the effectiveness of nursing and medical interventions in achieving established client care goals

7. Revise nursing interventions if goals have not been achieved

DESCRIPTION

A cerebral vascular accident, which is commonly referred to as a stroke, occurs when the blood supply to the brain is diminished through vascular occlusion or rupture of a blood vessel.[12,13] There are several types of "stroke".

Transient Cerebral Ischemic Attack

Transient cerebral ischemic attack (TIA) is the term used

to describe "little strokes, " in which ischemia to the cerebral tissue is temporary, lasting only a few minutes to 24 hours; there are no noticeable residual effects.

Transient Cerebral Ischemic Attack-Incomplete Recovery

Transient cerebral ischemic attack-incomplete recovery (TIA-IR) is another type of attack which may last for several days and leaves the client with some minor residual effects.

Completed Stroke

Completed stroke (CS) is the diagnosis made when the attack of cerebral ischemia presents more severe stroke symptoms; the onset is abrupt and partial or complete recovery is made. [12]

Approximately 200, 000 people die from CVA each year.

ETIOLOGY

The three main causes of CVA are:

1. Cerebral embolism

2. Cerebral thrombosis

3. Cerebral hemorrhage [5, 12]

The cerebral embolism may consist of air, fat, a small portion of a thrombus that has settled in the cerebral vessel, tumor, or bacterial clumps. [5, 12]

Cerebral thrombosis is the most common cause of stroke.[12] Illnesses predisposing to cerebral thrombosis include: arteriosclerosis, syphilis and other infections, dehydration, and trauma. [5]

Cerebral hemorrhage usually is caused by the rupture of a cerebral vessel affected by arteriosclerosis or weakened by an aneurysm or hypertension.[5, 12] Stroke from cerebral hemorrhage usually produces more extensive neurologic defects and recovery is slower. Other less frequent causes of stroke include: recurrent ischemic attacks, hypertensive encephalopathy, migrainous hemiplegia, and syncope. [5]

ASSESSMENT SPECIFIC TO THE ALTERATION

Subjective Data (Symptoms)

The client experiencing a thrombus-caused CVA usually has had previous transient ischemic attacks (TIAs). Some of the forewarning symptoms include:

Attacks of falling down or dropping things

Blurring of vision

Transient blindness in one eye

Transient paresthesias

Ataxia

Dysphagia

Nerve palsies

Disorientation

Dizziness or lightheadedness

Changes in behavior[9]

The symptoms of a cerebral vascular accident are variable depending on the etiology, location of the ischemia, and the degree of damage that has occurred to the brain cells.[9,12] In cerebral hemorrhage and cerebral embolism, the onset of symptoms is usually abrupt. The onset of symptoms is more gradual in cerebral thrombosis because the occlusion of the blood vessel is more gradual.[12] Preliminary symptoms may be experienced such as headache, dizziness, mental confusion, poor coordination, and tingling sensations.[5,12]

Objective Data

A frequent nursing assessment of the client's neurologic status should include:

1. Level of consciousness

2. Vital signs

3. Pupillary changes

4. Movement and strength of extremities

5. Reflex status: deep reflexes (biceps, brachioradialis, triceps, patellar, Achilles); superficial reflexes (upper abdominal, lower abdominal, cremasteric, plantar, gluteal); and pathologic reflexes (Babinski, Chaddock, Oppenheim, Gordon)

6. Cranial nerves when possible

Cranial Nerve	Name
I	Olfactory
II	Optic
III	Oculomotor
IV	Trochlear
V	Trigeminal
VI	Abducens
VII	Facial
VIII	Acoustic
X	Glossopharyngeal
XI	Vagus
XI	Spinal Accessory
XII	Hypoglossal [9]

Any physical assessment text may be referred to for specific testing techniques. Neurologic symptoms are due to ischemia and include loss of sensation, hemiplegia, and reflex changes. If the left side of the brain is affected, right-sided paralysis of the face, arm, and leg will be present. Since the speech center for a right-handed person is located in the left side of the brain, aphasia also would be present if the left side of the brain was affected.[12] Emotional disturbances are common after a CVA. The onset could be sudden with loss of consciousness, convulsions, rapid and bounding pulse, labored or stertorous respirations, elevated blood pressure, and the pupils may not react to light normally. [16]

Late signs

Paralyzed limbs usually show signs of upper motor neuron disease: spastic weak muscles with little muscle atrophy, deep reflexes are hyperactive, superficial reflexes are decreased or absent and there is a positive Babinski sign. [5]

Diagnostic tests include:

1. Computerized axial tomography (CAT scan)

2. Cerebral angiography to detect aneurysms and vascular malformations or occlusions.

3. The EEG is abnormal in the majority of major CVAs.

4. The ECG may reveal the presence of a recent, silent myocardial infarction.

5. Other selected studies include skull films, pneumoencephalogram, and echoencephalography. [14]

CLIENT CARE GOALS

Medical and nursing interventions will be geared toward:

1. Maintaining and supporting the client's life processes

2. Preventing complications

3. Facilitating the client's adaptation to alterations in his biologic and psychologic state

4. Preventing future strokes [9]

INTERVENTIONS

During the acute phase of illness, interventions are aimed at keeping the client alive:

1. Maintaining a patent airway

2. Assessing the client's level of consciousness (recording the client's response to verbal and painful stimuli)

3. Evaluating vital signs for changes

4. Maintaining fluid and electrolyte balance

5. Performing a neurologic assessment at regular intervals to detect changes

Nursing support measures should be implemented to prevent complications such as contractures, decubiti, negative
nitrogen balance, vascular complications, atrophy of muscles
due to disuse, bladder distention, corneal irritation, self-injury
during convulsive seizures, infection, and respiratory complications. [1, 4]

In summary, general nursing interventions important in all
levels of consciousness include:

Maintaining an open   Verbal reassurance
   airway
                               Eye care
Oral hygiene
                               Skin care
Positioning
                               Nutrition
Exercise
                               Contacting the spiritual
Elimination   advisor for the client
                                  and family [13]

After the client regains consciousness, he will require an
orientation to time, place, and person. [1] Family and close
friends should be encouraged to participate in the reorientation
phase. If the client is aphasic, a means of communication
must be established. The client and his family will need a
great deal of emotional support as the neurologic deficits become more evident. Clients often experience periods of depression, frustration, irritability, denial, and anger. [14]

Rehabilitative interventions which were begun shortly after
admission, when the client's condition stabilized, are continued
more intensely with the following goals in mind:

1. Prevention of deformities

2. Retraining of the affected limbs

3. Assisting the client to gain independence in performing activities of daily living (eating, dressing, personal hygiene, walking)

4. Preparing the client and family for discharge 1, 4

Prior to discharge, the client and family should be taught some of the risk factors in stroke, so that a second stroke may be prevented. Prestroke risk factors include: obesity, poor nutrition, heredity, excessively stressful lifestyle, excessive smoking, and lack of exercise. [14]

Clients with the following conditions are considered to be in the high-risk category:

Atherosclerosis	ECG changes
Hypertension	Rheumatic heart disease
Arrhythmia	Diabetes mellitus
Ischemia	Hypercholesteremia
Gout	Postural hypotension
Cardiomegaly	Myocardial infarction [14]

MEDICAL INTERVENTIONS

The medical management of cerebrovascular disease is highly individualized and controversial. Winkelman states that anticoagulation and carotid endarterectomy are widely used in clients experiencing transient ischemic attacks. [19] Anticoagulation with heparin followed by warfarin (Coumadin) and placing the client on limited activity appear to be significantly effective in preventing subsequent cerebral infarction. [2,19] There is some disagreement among physicians as to whether TIAs associated with unilateral carotid stenosis are benefited by carotid surgery. [2] Therapeutic results also have been obtained by using anticoagulants in clients experiencing "stroke in evolution" or "evolving stroke"; acute anticoagulation may lessen the final neurologic deficit. [2,19] In completed stroke, the treatment is largely supportive. [2]

Cerebral infarction secondary to embolism sometimes is treated by anticoagulation if the spinal fluid is clear, [2]

although there have been some reports that hemorrhagic infarction may be produced by immediate anticoagulation.[2] Medical treatment of the client experiencing intracerebral or subarachnoid hemorrhage is dependent upon the etiology and the
location.

General measures include:

1. Bed rest.

2. Sedation in alert clients.

3. Control of cerebral edema (mannitol 20% IV, dexameth-
   asone IV, hyperventilation).

4. Antifibrinolytic therapy with aminocaproic acid (Amicar)
   is useful in subarachnoid hemorrhage due to ruptured
   aneurysm.

5. Control of hypertension.

6. Stool softeners to prevent straining at stool.[2]

Central nervous system depressant drugs should be avoided.

The rehabilitative program for clients whose only disabi-
lity is hemiplegia is divided into four phases and is under the
direction of the physical therapist:

1. The bed phase starts the second or third day after the
   onset, when the client is conscious; exercises are begun using the overhead trapeze mechanism starting
   with 10 minutes of exercise every 4 hours and increased
   daily; the client does self-care with the uninvolved
   hand (personal hygiene, feeding).

2. The standing phase starts 3 to 5 days after the beginning of the bed phase; the client continues exercises
   to rise to a standing position, does slight knee bends,
   up on toes, and sitting down; self-care continues.

3. The stair-climbing phase usually starts 2 to 10 days
   after the client begins the standing phase, self-care
   continues, some bracing may be prescribed.

4. In the cane-walking phase the cane is held in the unaffected hand; the client learns slow gait and then fast
gait. 5

If aphasia has occurred, speech therapy should be prescribed and initiated as soon as possible. 5

COMPLICATIONS

Decubitus ulcers, pneumonia, contractures, thrombosis,
kidney stones, urinary tract infections, orthopedic deformities
(foot and wrist drop) are all possible. 12

REVIEW QUESTIONS

1. What are the three main causes of stroke or cardiovascular
accident (CVA)?

2. Which of the three named in question 1 is considered to be
the most common cause?

3. Name at least four illnesses which predispose a person to
cerebral thrombosis.

4. List at least 10 forewarning symptoms of CVA.

5. A frequent nursing assessment of the client's neurologic
status should be done when the client has experienced a
CVA. Name six items that should be included in the neurologic assessment.

6. If the left side of the brain has been affected by the cerebral
vascular accident, which side of the body would you expect
to be paralyzed?

7. If a right-handed person experiences a CVA and the left
side of the brain is affected, would aphasia be present?

8. During the acute phase of illness, nursing support measures
are implemented to prevent complications. Name 10 complications that may occur if preventive measures are not
taken.

9. The rehabilitative program for hemiplegic clients can be
divided into four phases: bed phase, standing phase stair-
climbing phase, and cane-walking phase. Briefly explain
each phase.

10. Name at least <u>six</u> long-term complications due to prolonged bed rest.

REFERENCES

1. Beyers, M. and Dudas, S.: <u>The Clinical Practice of Medical-Surgical Nursing</u>. Boston: Little, Brown and Co., 1977, pp. 950-955.

2. Boedeker, E. and Dauber, J.: <u>Manual of Medical Therapeutics</u>. 21st Ed., Boston: Little, Brown and Co., 1974, pp. 396-398.

3. Breunig, K. A.: After the Blowup – How to Care for the Patient With A Ruptured Cerebral Aneurysm. <u>Nursing 76</u> (December 1976): 37-45.

4. Brunner, L. and Suddarth, D.: <u>The Lippincott Manual of Nursing Practice</u>. 2nd Ed., Philadelphia: J.B. Lippincott Co., 1978, pp. 912-918.

5. Chusid, J. C.: Nervous System. In Krupp, M.A. and Chatton, M.J.: <u>Current Medical Diagnosis and Treatment</u>. Los Altos, Calif.: Lange Medical Publications, pp. 566-570.

6. Dayhoff, N.: Re-Thinking Stroke: Soft or Hard Devices to Position Hands? <u>Am J Nurs</u> 75 (July 1975): 1142-1144.

7. Fowler, R. and Fordyce, W. E.: <u>Stroke: Why Do They Behave That Way</u>? Washington State Heart Association, 1974.

8. Goldberg, R.L. et al.: The Stroke Unit: Psychological Aspects of Recovery. <u>Psychosomatics</u> 20 (May 1979): 316-317.

9. Hudak, C. et al.: <u>Critical Care Nursing</u>. 2nd Ed., Philadelphia: J.B. Lippincott Co., 1977, pp. 451-462.

10. Mahoney, F. and Bartel, D.: <u>Up and Around</u>. Washington, D.C.: U.S. Department of Health, Education, and Welfare, Public Health Publication 1120.

11. McCormick, G. and Williams, M.: Stroke: The Double Crisis. <u>Am J Nurs</u> 79 (August 1979): 1410-1411.

12. Miller, B. and Keane, C.: Encyclopedia and Dictionary of Medicine, Nursing and Allied Health. 2nd Ed., Philadelphia: W. B. Saunders Co., 1978, pp. 192-195.

13. Murray, R. et al.: The Nursing Process in Later Maturity. Englewood Cliffs, NJ: Prentice-Hall, Inc., 1980. pp. 424-451.

14. Riehl, J. and Chambers, J.: Better Salvage For the Sroke Victim. Nursing 76 (July 1976): 24-31.

15. Ring, B. A.: An Overview: Computed Axial Tomography. Radiology 8 (November-December 1979): 110-112.

16. Shafer, K. et al.: Medical-Surgical Nursing. 6th Ed., St. Louis: C. V. Mosby Co., 1975, pp. 892-899.

17. Strike Back at Stroke. Distributed by the American Heart Association with permission of Chronic Disease Program, Public Health Service, U. S. Department of Health, Education, and Welfare. No. 50-024A.

18. Weisburg, J.: Doppler Today. Appl Radiol 9 (January-February 1980): 99-100.

19. Winkleman, A. C.: The Aggressive Management of the Stroke Patient. In Oaks, W. (Ed.): Critical Care Medicine. New York: Grune and Stratton, 1974, pp. 389-396.

CHAPTER 14

CONGESTIVE HEART FAILURE

LEARNING OBJECTIVES

Study of this chapter will enable the reader to:

1. Discuss the etiology of left and right ventricular heart failure

2. Detect the symptoms of left or right ventricular failure

3. Describe common physical findings related to left ventricular failure

4. Describe common physical findings related to right ventricular failure

5. Formulate individualized client care goals for the client experiencing congestive heart failure (CHF)

6. Plan specific nursing interventions to promote the client's physical and mental rest

7. Assess the client's understanding of the disease process and prescribed therapies

8. Design a teaching plan to assist the client in recognizing the signs of systemic and pulmonary fluid accumulation

9. Evaluate the effectiveness of health teaching by other health team members in regard to disease process, dietary alterations, medications, stress reduction, discharge planning, and prevention of exacerbation of the alteration

DESCRIPTION

Congestive heart failure (CHF) occurs when the heart is unable to pump an adequate volume of blood, which was received from the veins, to various body tissues to meet their metabolic demands.[10] In other words, cardiac output is reduced and the "supply does not equal the demand." Congestive heart failure sometimes is referred to as "pump failure." Following the decrease in myocardial contractility, there is sodium and water retention and an elevation of the pressure in the left atrium, which results in pulmonary vascular congestion.[3,10] Initially, only the left ventricle or the right ventricle may fail, but ultimately, combined failure of both ventricles is generally the rule.[10] Congestive heart failure may be present as an acute or chronic condition.

ETIOLOGY

In general, the basic causes of ventricular failure are:

1. Myocardial weakness or inflammation

2. Excessive work load due to:

    a. increased resistance to ejection

    b. increased stroke volume

    c. increased bodily demands[10]

More specifically, the etiology of left ventricular failure is commonly due to: hypertension, coronary artery disease, or valvular heart disease (aortic valvular disease is more common than mitral valvular disease).[10] Other less common causes of left ventricular failure include: hypertrophic cardiomyopathy, congenital heart lesions, left-to-right shunts, and congestive cardiomyopathies.[10]

The etiology of right ventricular failure is commonly due to mitral stenosis with increased pulmonary resistance, pulmonary parenchymal or vascular disease, or pulmonary valvular stenosis.[9,10] Less common causes of right ventricular failure include: tricuspid valvular disease or infective endocarditis, where the right side of the heart is involved.[10] Precipitating diseases or factors which increase the work load of the heart include:

Arrhythmias   Anemia

Respiratory infection   Excessive salt intake

Myocardial infarction	Corticosteroid administration
Pulmonary embolism	Pregnancy
Rheumatic carditis	Excessive or rapid adminis- tration of intravenous fluids [10]
Thyrotoxicosis	

ASSESSMENT SPECIFIC TO THE ALTERATION

Signs and symptoms are variable depending on whether the failure is unilateral or bilateral (both right and left failure) and the degree of failure present.[11] Initially, there may be unilateral ventricular failure, but in time the other ventricle will fail due to the increased work load thrust upon it.[3] Symptoms of both right and left failure can occur simultaneously.[1]

LEFT VENTRICULAR FAILURE

Subjective Data

The client experiencing left ventricular failure will frequently complain of:

1. Exertional dyspnea

2. Orthopnea

3. Paroxysmal nocturnal dyspnea

4. Cough

5. Restlessness

6. Palpitations

7. Exertional fatigue and weakness (late symptoms)

8. Decreased urinary output [4, 5, 10, 11]

Objective Data

If overt right ventricular failure is absent, physical examination by the physician should disclose the following:

1. The basic cause of the left ventricular failure (e.g.,
   myocardial infarction, hypertension, valvular disease
   (aortic or mitral).

2. Left ventricular hypertrophy: apical impulse is forceful (or heaving) and is displaced to the left and downward; these findings may be confirmed by the chest
   x-ray and electrocardiogram.

3. Radiologic evidence of pulmonary venous distention
   and possibly hydrothorax.

4. Basilar rales which do not clear on coughing may be
   present.

5. Other signs may be present such as S3 ventricular gallop rhythm, pulsus alternans (a succession of alternating strong and weak beats), P2 is accentuated, and
   there are behavioral changes.[10]

Left ventricular failure may progress to acute pulmonary
edema. The client experiences severe dyspnea and anxiety.
Other signs are: cyanosis, tachycardia, diaphoresis, pro-
ductive cough (frothy, pink-tinged sputum), crackling rales,
and diminished or absent breath sounds in various lobes, depending on the extent of pulmonary edema.[10, 11]

RIGHT VENTRICULAR FAILURE

The signs and symptoms are predominantly those of elevated pressures and congestion in the systemic veins and capillaries.[3]

Subjective Data

The client often complains of: unexplained weight gain,
nausea and vomiting, anorexia, weakness, and nocturia.[3, 11]

Objective Data

Signs of right ventricular failure include:

Engorgement of the neck veins

Edema of the ankles (may be the pitting type)

Ascites

Hepatomegaly

Pericardial effusion

Pleural effusion

Weakness

In severe cases, changes in mentation [3, 10, 11]

Laboratory tests reveal:

1. High specific gravity, significant proteinuria and granular casts in the urine.

2. The BUN (blood urea nitrogen) level may be elevated.

3. Serum levels of sodium, potassium, and carbon dioxide are within normal limits before diuretics are used.[10]

Diagnostic tests include: electrocardiogram, chest x-ray, arterial blood gas studies, and liver function studies. [3]

CLIENT CARE GOALS

1. The etiology of the client's congestive heart failure will be identified and corrected or removed.

2. Cardiac function will be improved through the use of therapeutic interventions which will: increase the force and efficiency of myocardial contraction and reduce the cardiac work load.

3. Educate the client regarding the disease process, signs of decompensation, prescribed medications (name, dosage, action, toxic effects, interactions), prescribed diet, reduction or elimination of risk factors which place an excessive work load on the heart.

4. Plan and implement health measures to prevent the recurrence of congestive heart failure and therefore improve the quality of his/her life.[10, 11]

INTERVENTIONS

General interventions for the client experiencing congestive heart failure include:

Mental and physical rest	Diuretic therapy
Comfortably cool environment	Fluid restriction, if appropriate
Reduction in dietary sodium	Supportive measures
A digitalis preparation	Client education [2, 4, 10, 11]

Rest

Physical and mental rest can reduce the cardiac work load; decreasing the metabolic activity decreases the need for oxygen. Nursing interventions to promote this goal are:

1. Planning activities to conserve the client's energy(i.e., anticipating the client's needs, putting essential items within easy reach, etc.)

2. Providing adequate rest periods.

3. Positioning the client comfortably: a sitting position is often preferred by the client and it has the added advantage of reducing venous return to the heart and lungs, therefore alleviating some of the client's symptoms.

4. Reducing the client's level of anxiety: oxygen administration may be necessary to diminish the work of
breathing and relieve any cerebral hypoxia that may
be present, listening while the client verbalizes his
needs, fears, etc., and answering the client's questions as intelligently and realistically as possible can
aid in reducing anxiety.

5. Relieving client's pain: caution and judgement should
be used when administering drugs, since congestive
heart failure may limit the detoxifying functions of
the liver.

6. Preventing the hazards of immobility (i.e., decubitus
ulcers, pulmonary congestion, pulmonary embolism)
by using frequent massage, position changes, alternating pressure mattress, deep-breathing exercises,
leg exercises, and elastic stockings. [1, 3]

Diet

A reduction in dietary sodium intake is frequently prescribed by the physician to rid the body of extracellular fluid
retention. The degree of sodium restriction depends on the
severity of the signs and symptoms, but severely restricted
sodium diets usually are not ordered for the client at home,
since he/she is often unable to comply with it. [11] Boedeker and
Dauber feel that most clients can be managed on a 2 g salt diet. [2]
The classification of sodium diets of the American Heart Association is:

250 mg sodium (0.6 g salt)

500 mg sodium (1.25 g salt)

750 mg sodium (1.9 g salt)

1000 mg sodium (2.5 g salt) [2]

The average daily dietary intake of sodium in the United States
is estimated at 6 to 15 g. [2, 11] Clients usually are told not
to add salt to their food at the table and to avoid using it during
cooking preparation. Clients should be instructed to avoid:

Mineral water, club soda

Bicarbonate and other sodium-containing medications

Canned soups and vegetables

Salad dressings

Canned fish

Cheese

Cured and smoked ham, sausages

Pickles

Nuts

Crackers and prepared cereals except wheat, oatmeal, puffed wheat and rice, Instant Ralston, and shredded wheat

Excessive milk ingestion [2]

Several salt substitutes are available, but should only be used after obtaining the physician's approval. The dietitian is usually responsible for instructing the client regarding diet, however, the nurse should reinforce what has been taught and assess whether or not the client understands his prescribed diet.

Medication

A digitalis preparation usually is indicated in clients experiencing CHF. Digitalis has positive inotropic effects on the myocardium. Actions of digitalis include:

1. It stimulates the vagus nerve and the ventricular myocardium.

2. It inhibits transmission of the impulse from the atrium to the ventricles, resulting in a slower heart rate, a stronger systolic contraction, an increased cardiac output, and more complete emptying of the ventricles.[6]

Because the blood supply to the kidneys is increased, diuresis also occurs and edema is relieved.[3, 6] There are several preparations on the market for oral and parenteral administration. Digitoxin and digoxin are commonly used oral or intravenous preparations. Deslanoside (Cedilanid-D) and ouabain are parenteral preparations. The choice of drug is dependent on the speed of onset, duration of action, personal

preference of the physician, and whether renal or hepatic failure is present.[3,11] Digitoxin is excreted by the liver; therefore, if the client has hepatic failure, this drug would not be used.
The effects of digitoxin may last for 2 to 3 weeks. A digitali-
zing dose of digitoxin may vary from 1 to 1.5 mg; a maintenance dose of digitoxin might range from 0.05 to 0.2 mg.[6,11]

Digoxin is excreted by the kidney. The oral digitilizing
dose of digoxin varies from 2.0 to 4.0 mg; the maintenance dose
may be 0.125 to 0.75 mg depending on the serum levels of
digoxin.[6] The effect of digoxin is completely gone in 2 to 6
days.[11] Onset of action is more rapid for digoxin than digitoxin.[4] The margin of safety with digitalis between side effects
and toxicity is narrow.

There are numerous side effects, but anorexia usually precedes nausea and vomiting by a day or two.[4] Toxic effects include:

1. Gastrointestinal effects: anorexia, nausea, vomiting,
    diarrhea, copious salivation, abdominal discomfort.

2. Cardiac effects: very slow radial pulse due to heart
    block or arrhythmias; arrhythmias of many types may
    occur as well as premature ventricular contractions.

3. Neurologic effects (may occur early): headache, ver-
    tigo, fatigue, drowsiness, depression, confusion,
    aphasia, disorientation, neuralgic pain in the lower
    one-third of the face may occur.

4. Visual effects: blurred vision, halos, changes in color
    vision

5. Skin rashes and eosinophilia are rare.

6. Gynecomastia may occur in men.[11]

It is especially important that the nurse monitor the client's
serum potassium level, since a decrease in this level poten-
tiates the action of digitalis and increases the risk of cardiotoxicity.[11] Potassium supplements may be administered if
needed.

Propranolol has a negative inotropic effect on the heart
and extreme caution should be used when administering it to
clients with congestive heart failure. The nurse administering

a digitalis preparation must be sure to obtain an apical and radial pulse rate for 1 full minute before administering the drug.
(Traditionally, if the pulse rate was 60 or less, the physician
was notified before administering it; more recently, physicians
are setting a lower pulse rate at which they wish to be informed.)
The client should be observed for other signs of digitalis intoxication.

   Diuretics are frequently prescribed to enhance the excretion of sodium and water in clients experiencing congestive
heart failure. Diuretics have the ability to impair the tubular
absorption of sodium, but they do not eliminate the underlying
causative factors which initially led to the extracellular fluid
load.[11] Common diuretic agents are ethacrynic acid, furosemide, hydrochlorothiazide, and spironolactone. (These agents
can be reviewed in the Appendix of this text.) The client should
be weighed daily to determine if edema is being controlled; intake and output should also be carefully recorded.[3]

Education

   The nurse working cooperatively with the physician can
play an important role in client education. A teaching plan
must be developed to meet the individual client's needs and
should consider the client's intellectual abilities, motivation
to learn, cultural background and social situation. The client's
family should be invited to participate in the teaching-learning
process.

   The nurse can facilitate the client's adaptation to illness
by helping him understand the disease process. Most authorities agree that the term "failure" can be very frightening to
the client and his family. It should be explained that the term
failure does not mean a complete and irreversible process.[11]
Illustrations of the heart's structure and function can be utilized
to facilitate understanding. Explanations should be made in
terminology that the client and his family can understand; medical jargon can confuse the client and family and only increases
their level of anxiety. The client must be able to recognize
the signs of cardiac decompensation. Long lists of signs and
symptoms are often difficult to remember. Waxler[11] suggests
having the client describe how he felt when he first became ill;
this should help him to remember the signs and symptoms, and
that they should be reported if they occur.

Systemic and pulmonary fluid accumulation must be recognized by the client. He should be taught to look for and report:

An increase in weight (2 to 3 lbs in 1 or 2 days)

Swelling of the ankles

Shoes or clothes becoming more tight

Recurrent cough

Tiredness

Slowing down in general [11]

Daily weights should be done before eating breakfast, after voiding, and with the client dressed in similar type clothes. [11]

In regard to medications, the client and family should know the name, precise dosage, route of administration, and toxic effects of the prescribed drugs. Clients taking digitalis preparations should be taught to take their pulse, at rest, before taking the medication. A rate below 60 or above 100 beats per minute or any change in regularity should be reported to the physician.

Dietary alterations can be reviewed and reinforced by the nurse. The client should be encouraged to verbalize any concerns regarding the prescribed dietary changes. The physician should be consulted regarding the use of a salt substitute.

The client should be made aware of how physical exertion, emotional stress, and infections affect the heart's function. Activities that cause dyspnea or emotional stress should be avoided. [11] Consideration should be given to obtaining "flu" immunizations. The client should seek medical assistance whenever other illnesses occur. [11] Daily activities should be resumed gradually or as directed by the client's physician.

COMPLICATIONS

Pulmonary edema, pulmonary embolization, pulmonary infections, cardiac cirrhosis, peripheral arterial embolization, and electrolyte disturbances are common complications. [10]

REVIEW QUESTIONS

1. Is congestive heart failure an acute or chronic condition?

2. List the common causes of left and right ventricular failure.

3. Is congestive heart failure a unilateral or bilateral condition?

4. Can symptoms of both right and left failure occur simultaneously?

5. Name seven symptoms of left ventricular failure.

6. List eight signs of acute pulmonary edema.

7. Name five symptoms of right ventricular failure.

8. Name eight signs of right ventricular failure.

9. There are many factors which can place an excessive work load on the heart. Name at least three common ones.

10. Describe six nursing interventions aimed at promoting physical and mental rest.

11. Give the rationale for reducing dietary sodium intake.

12. Name at least ten foods that should be avoided when sodium restriction is prescribed.

13. What are the effects of digitalis preparations on the myocardium?

14. Which digitalis preparation should be avoided if the client has hepatic failure?

15. What side effects may occur when a digitalis preparation is administered?

16. What effect does propranolol have on the heart?

17. Name six common complications of congestive heart failure.

REFERENCES

1. Beyers, M. and Dudas, S.: The Clinical Practice of Medical-Surgical Nursing. Boston: Little, Brown, and Co., 1977, pp. 375-383.

2. Boedeker, E. and Dauber, J.: Manual of Medical Therapeutics. 21st Ed., Boston: Little, Brown, and Co., 1974, pp. 101-117.

3. Brunner, L. and Suddarth, D.: The Lippincott Manual of Nursing Practice. 2nd Ed., Philadelphia: J.B. Lippincott Co., 1978, pp. 368-375.

4. Burch, G.: Cardiac Edema. Consultant 20 (April 1980): 227-232.

5. Cohen, S.: New Concepts in Understanding Congestive Heart Failure. Part I: How the Clinical Features Arise. Am J Nurs 81 (January 1981): 119-142.

6. Falconer, M. et al.: The Drug-The Nurse-The Patient. 6th Ed., Philadelphia: W.B. Saunders Co., 1978, pp. 301-309.

7. Giles, T. D.: Principles of Vasodilator Therapy for Left Ventricular Congestive Heart Failure. Heart Lung 9 (March-April 1980): 271-276.

8. Greco, F. del: The Kidney in Congestive Heart Failure. Mod Conc Cardiovasc Dis 44 (September 1975): 47-52.

9. Hurst, K.: A Major Set-Back. Nurs Mirror 150 (February 7, 1980): 38-40.

10. Sokolow, M.: Heart and Great Vessels. In Krupp, M.A. and Chatton, M.J.: Current Medical Diagnosis and Treatment. Los Altos Calif.: Lange Medical Publications, 1976, pp. 213-222.

11. Waxler, R.: The Patient With Congestive Heart Failure. Nurs Clin N Am 11 (June 1976): 297-308.

12. Winslow, E. H. (Ed.): Teaching and Rehabilitating the Cardiac Patient. Nurs Clin N Am 11 (June 1976): 211-383.

CHAPTER 15

HYPERTENSION

LEARNING OBJECTIVES

Study of this chapter will enable the reader to:

1. Define the term "hypertension" as accepted by the World Health Organization

2. Discuss the circulatory factors influencing arterial pressure

3. Explain the difference between primary (essential) hypertension and secondary hypertension

4. Discuss the various theories of causation being explored in relation to hypertension

5. Identify the target organs or systems affected by sustained, uncontrolled hypertension

6. Employ effective interviewing techniques in obtaining historical data

7. Describe the method to be used for accurate blood pressure determination

8. Use appropriate physical assessment techniques when assessing the client with hypertension

9. Describe diagnostic examinations to rule out secondary causes of hypertension

10. Describe the importance of nonpharmacologic therapies in blood pressure control

11. Discuss the pharmacologic agents available for blood pressure control, citing usual dosages, mechanism of action, and side effects

12. Formulate a plan to educate the client in regard to diet alterations, rest, exercise, medications, relaxation techniques, and the importance of health care follow-up visits

DESCRIPTION

The World Health Organization accepts the following criteria in defining hypertension: A persistent elevation of the systolic blood pressure above 140 mm Hg and of the diastolic pressure above 90 mm Hg.[17,29] A single elevated blood pressure reading does not establish a diagnosis of hypertension. Stress, anxiety, any discomfort, and physical activity all cause a sharp elevation in blood pressure, but the elevation is transient.[16] Several of the circulatory factors that influence arterial pressure are:

Cardiac output

Peripheral resistance

Blood volume

Viscosity of the blood

Elasticity of the arteries [2]

Peripheral resistance in the arterioles is often increased in hypertension, but cardiac output may be normal.[16] Any factors (drugs, hormones, etc.) which cause stimulation of the sympathetic nerves of the smooth muscle layers of the arterioles will be responsible for constriction of the arterioles and therefore increase peripheral resistance.[2]

Classification

Hypertension may be classified as:

1. Primary hypertension (essential hypertension) which accounts for approximately 85 to 90% of the cases.

2. Secondary hypertension which accounts for approximately 10 to 15% of the cases.

Hypertension may be further subclassified as:

1. Mild: diastolic pressure usually 90 to 114 mm Hg

2. Moderate: diastolic usually 115 to 129 mm Hg

3. Severe: diastolic pressure greater than 130 mm Hg [3]

Classifications are variable depending on the resources consulted. Hypertension often is referred to as the "silent killer" because of its insidious onset. [2]

ETIOLOGY

The exact etiology of primary hypertension is unknown; however, several theories of causation are being explored which include:

1. Hypersensitive sympathetic vasoconstricting nerves

2. Psychogenic factors

3. Hormonal imbalance

4. Hereditary tendency

5. Renin-angiotensin-aldosterone system

6. A combination of several factors [4, 17]

Secondary hypertension follows some other pathologic conditions such as:

1. Renal disease: renal vascular occlusion, polycystic renal disease, glomerulonephritis, or polynephritis

2. Coarctation of the aorta

3. Endocrine disturbances: pheochromocytoma, tumors of the adrenal cortex, or Cushing syndrome

4. Eclampsia [2, 4, 17]

Women who have been taking oral contraceptive agents also display a secondary type of hypertension. The precise reason for this is not known, but it is speculated that the sodium and water retaining effects of these agents are responsible for the increased fluid volume and increased blood pressure. The diagnosis of primary hypertension is reached only after secondary causes of hypertension have been ruled out by physical examination and laboratory studies. [16]

ASSESSMENT SPECIFIC TO THE ALTERATION

Historical data collection is extremely important. The nurse must utilize effective interviewing techniques to obtain information which is accurate, concise, and pertinent to the client's health status. The interview offers an opportunity to assess the client's psychologic responses to his health alteration, as well as his biologic responses. Acceptance of the alteration may be especially difficult if the client has been asymptomatic up to the time of diagnosis. Historical data collection "specific" to the client who has or is suspected of having hypertension should include information regarding:

Family history of hypertension	Birth control pills or other medications
Previous personal history of hypertension	Personal habits such as cigarette smoking and alcohol consumption
Hyperlipidemia	Daily pattern of activity (exercise)
Amount of daily salt intake	
Ingestion of black licorice	Ability to deal with stressful situations[4]

A complete physical examination should follow the collection of historical data. Careful blood pressure determinations should be done with the client in three different positions: (1) supine, (2) sitting, and (3) standing.

Both arms should be used to get baseline data. It is important to use the proper size blood pressure cuff. Generally, a cuff width for the obese client should be 18 to 20 cm in width (or 20% wider than the diameter of the limb); cuff width for the nonobese client is usually 12 to 14 cm wide. [1, 9] When recording the blood pressure, include the client's position during the measurement and indicate the extremity used. All vital signs should be assessed. The ophthalmoscopic examination is very important in detecting vascular changes in the small blood vessels, such as hemorrhage, exudates, tortuosity, or narrowing of the blood vessels. The heart and peripheral pulses should be examined. The point of maximum impulse (PMI) should be palpated and described along with other heart sounds and murmurs, if present. Auscultation over peripheral arteries and the abdomen should be done to detect bruits, if present. A neurologic screening test should be done to detect any neurologic deficits. The technique of a complete physical examination may be found in any physical assessment text. It should be remembered that only a portion of the client's assessment specific to the hypertensive client is presented here. Total client assessment will require exploration of all biologic systems, as well as psychologic responses.

Subjective Data (Symptoms) and Objective Data (Signs) in Relation to the Specific Types of Hypertension

Primary Hypertension

The client may be asymptomatic or may complain of a morning occipital headache. If more symptoms are present, they are usually nonspecific and related to the complications of the disease (cardiovascular, cerebral, or renal in origin). [4] The diastolic blood pressure is "persistently" greater than 90 mm Hg and the systolic blood pressure is greater than 140 mm Hg. Other objective data would depend on the organ system involved. [4, 17]

Malignant Hypertension

This is an accelerated phase of hypertension, which occurs in a small percentage of persons with primary hypertension. [16] Blood pressure levels are extremely high in this alteration, but the diagnosis is not made by the blood pressure alone. [18] The diagnosis is based on the degree of papilledema of the optic disc and on urinary findings. [18]

Subjective data include: visual impairment, morning headache, weight loss, dizziness, nausea, and vomiting.

Objective data collection includes:

Proteinuria.

Microscopic hematuria.

Plasma renin activity.

Ophthalmoscopic examination reveals papilledema, retinopathy, hemorrhages, and exudates.

Lowered specific gravity.

An increased blood urea nitrogen (BUN) of more than 100 mg/100 ml blood, which suggests renal involvement.

Usually, the diastolic pressure is greater than 120 mm Hg.

Progressive renal insufficiency follows. [4, 14]

Secondary Hypertension

Subjective data: the client may complain of headache, palpitations, tremor, weight loss, and excessive sweating.

Objective data collection reveals:

Symptomatic paroxysms of hypertension (usually less than 1 year)

Tachycardia

Hypertensive retinopathy

Hypermetabolism

Increased fasting blood sugar

Excretion of catecholamines in the urine [19]

Clients with renovascular hypertension may give a history of hematuria, renal trauma, dyspnea, or acute flank pain. Objective data include:

Systolic and diastolic bruit in the epigastrium or upper quadrants.

Intravenous pyelogram is abnormal.

There is a decrease in urine and sodium output.

Fluid retention.

Edema.[17,19]

The client with primary aldosteronism may complain of muscular weakness, polyuria, nocturia, polydipsia, paresthesias, and headache. Objective data include:

Moderate elevation of the blood pressure

Tetany

Dilute alkaline urine, and persistenly low serum potassium levels (below 3. 5 mEq/L), urinary potassium is greater than 40 mEq/24 hr[17]

When the client has coarctation of the aorta, the complaint may be weight loss. Objective data include:

Absence of femoral pulses

Decreased blood pressure in the legs when compared to the arms

Notching of the ribs on x-ray

Intercostal bruits on auscultation[17]

Objective data for the client who has Cushing syndrome include:

Mild hypertension

Moon facies

"Buffalo hump" on back

Edema

Hirsutism

Excretion of large amounts of 17-hydroxycorticoids and 17-ketosteroids in the urine[17, 19]

DIAGNOSTIC EXAMINATIONS

Secondary causes of hypertension can usually be ruled out by physical examination and laboratory studies such as:

Serum electrolytes	Creatinine
Urinalysis	Blood sugars
Complete blood count	Blood uric acid
Blood urea nitrogen	Chest x-ray
Electrocardiography	Intravenous pyelogram
Serum cholesterol	Serum triglycerides[6]

More specific tests are available if pheochromocytoma, primary aldosteronism, Cushing syndrome, or renal disease is suspected. It is beyond the scope of this book to deal with these numerous tests.

CLIENT CARE GOALS

General client care goals to consider:

1. Blood pressure reduction to normotensive or acceptable levels.

2. Blood pressure reduction will be maintained with minimum therapeutic side effects.

3. Risk factors will be identified and reduced.

4. Pathologic progression of the disease will be delayed.

5. Client's lifestyle will be altered in such a way that it is both acceptable to the client and family and compatible with established health care goals.

6. The disease process and the complications which arise from uncontrolled hypertension will be understood by the client and family.

7. Responsibility for personal health care will be assumed by the client.

8. Continued regular health care follow-up will be available and accepted by the client. [4, 7, 17]

INTERVENTIONS

Interventions are determined on an individual basis and are influenced by the type of hypertension the client has, the degree of blood pressure elevation, and the extent of complications due to the progression of the disease. Interventions are directed toward the accomplishment of established client care goals.

Education

Client education is extremely important regardless of the therapeutic regimen prescribed. This intervention is often executed by the nurse, but client education is the responsibilty of all health team members. An educated client is more apt to be compliant in following the established therapeutic regimen. The client who has been asymptomatic, but develops side effects to the prescribed drugs, may be more likely to continue taking the drugs if he understands the disease process and the outcomes if hypertension is left uncontrolled. The nurse should assess the client's level of knowledge regarding hypertension and the therapeutic regimen, readiness to learn about hypertension (includes level of anxiety), motivation for learning, as well as the client's psychosocial adaptation to illness.[1] Once the learning needs have been identified, the nurse and the client can collaborate on establishing goals for learning more about hypertension and the prescribed therapeutic regimen.

Therapy

If the client has mild hypertension, conservative therapy may be instituted initially. Generally, this involves some alterations in lifestyle such as:

Weight reduction, if the client is obese, to decrease the workload of the heart

Decreased sodium intake to decrease the plasma volume

Improvement of physical condition through progressive exercise

Identification of major psychologic stresses

Elimination or reduction of cigarette smoking

Decreased fat intake in the diet [4, 13]

Medication

The alterations in lifestyle may not be adequate to control the hypertension and many physicians feel that some form of drug therapy will be needed if:

1. The client's diastolic pressures are above 105 mm Hg.

2. Damage to the target organs is present.

3. The client has more than one of these risk factors: young age, black race, male, systolic greater than 160 mm Hg.

4. Positive family history of cardiovascular disease, hyperlipidemia, diabetes mellitus, or cigarette smoking.[13]

Initial drug therapy may include a single drug such as a thiazide diuretic or furosemide (Lasix), if the client has renal damage.[22] If the diuretic alone is ineffectual, a combination of drugs may be added. An adrenergic blocker such as reserpine, guanethidine, methyldopa, or clonidine may be added to the diuretic. If the combination does not produce the desired effect, a vasodilator such as hydralazine and a beta-blocker such as propranolol may be added to the diuretic and the adrenergic blocker.[13] Metoprolol (Lopressor), a cardioselective beta-blocker, is a newer medication recently approved for use in the United States.[22]

The nurse should assess the client's level of knowledge regarding his drug regimen. The client should be fully oriented to the medications prescribed by the physician. The orientation should include the anticipated therapeutic effects of the medications, as well as their side effects. The client should be instructed to report any side effects of the drugs promptly.[2]

Common diuretics include: chlorothiazide (Diuril), hydrochlorothiazide (Esidrix, HydroDIURIL, Oretic), and chlorthalidone (Hygroton).

Stronger diuretics include: ethacrynic acid (Edecrin) and furosemide (Lasix).

(See the Appendix for usual adult dosages, mechanism of action, and common side effects.)

Other Interventions

Other nursing interventions include: educating the client in regard to diet alterations, avoiding the use of over-the-counter drugs without the physician's approval, alternatives to oral contraceptives, and the importance of adequate rest.[2]

Certain foods have been implicated in elevating the blood pressure and should be avoided. These include:

Pickled herring	Canned figs
Chocolate	Yeast products
Chicken liver	Beer and wine
Black licorice	Cheese (strong or aged) [2]

The client may be advised to include a banana or citrus fruit in his diet to help prevent potassium depletion, but supplementary potassium is often more effective when diuretics are being used daily. [2]

Selected clients may be taught to take their blood pressure at home. This is not recommended, if the client expresses undue anxiety regarding this. [2] When the client returns home, he may be instructed to record his daily weight, measure his abdominal girth, avoid obviously salty foods, and report any signs and symptoms of electrolyte imbalance. While the client is hospitalized, the nurse carefully monitors the blood pressure, electrolytes, various laboratory studies, and the client's total adaptive responses. If economic problems exist, the nurse should refer the client to the social worker or other health team member, who can assist with financial help.

Malignant hypertension is considered to be a medical emergency and requires prompt blood pressure reduction to reduce the client's risk of developing a stroke, cardiac failure, or renal failure. [14] Prolonged hypertensive states lead to blood vessel damage in the kidneys, pancreas, adrenal glands, and retina. [8] Drug therapy usually is begun promptly after a "brief" history and physical examination. [14] Since rapid blood pressure control is desired, parenteral agents are generally used. These drugs can be found in the Appendix under "Drugs Used in Hypertensive Emergencies. " These potent agents require that the nurse monitor the client constantly for major side effects, changes in vital signs, client's total response to therapy, and the condition of the intravenous site. Commonly used drugs that act directly on the vascular smooth muscle include: diazoxide (Hyperstat), sodium nitroprusside (Nipride), and hydralazine (Apresoline). Drugs which act on the sympathetic nervous system that also may be used include: trimethaphan (Arfonad), phentolamine (Regitine), methyldopa (Aldomet), and reserpine (Serpasil). [14]

Secondary forms of hypertension such as those caused by coarctation of the aorta, pheochromocytoma, primary aldosteronism, Cushing syndrome, and renal artery stenosis are amenable to surgical intervention. Nursing interventions would be dictated by the specific surgical procedure performed.

COMPLICATIONS

Sustained uncontrolled hypertension affects four target organs or systems:

1. Central nervous system response: headache, encephalopathy, cerebral hemorrhage, cerebrovascular accident

2. Eye response: papilledema, retinal vascular sclerosis, exudation, and hemorrhage

3. Cardiovascular response: left ventricular hypertrophy, congestive heart failure, angina pectoris, myocardial infarction, peripheral vascular disease

4. Genitourinary response: nephrosclerosis and eventual renal failure [4, 12, 25]

REVIEW QUESTIONS

1. Define hypertension as accepted by the World Health Organization.

2. Why is hypertension sometimes referred to as the "silent killer"?

3. Discuss the theories of causation in relation to primary hypertension.

4. Name at least four causes of secondary hypertension.

5. What are the three positions that should be used when determining the client's blood pressure.

6. Of what importance is the ophthalmoscopic examination?

7. What are the symptoms of primary hypertension? Explain your answer.

8. Name six symptoms of malignant hypertension.

9. List six signs of Cushing syndrome.

10. Discuss drug therapy in relation to hypertension.

11. Certain foods have been implicated in elevating the blood pressure. Name at least eight.

12. Sustained uncontrolled hypertension affects four target organs or systems. Name the four systems affected.

REFERENCES

1. Alderman, M. (Ed.): Hypertension: The Nurse's Role in Ambulatory Care. New York: Springer Publishing Co., 1977.

2. Beyers, M. and Dudas, S.: The Clinical Practice of Medical-Surgical Nursing. Boston: Little, Brown and Co., 1977, pp. 336-342.

3. Boediker, E. and Dauber, J.: Manual of Medical Therapeutics. 21st Ed., Boston: Little, Brown and Co., 1974. pp. 147-156.

4. Brunner, L. and Suddarth, D.: The Lippincott Manual of Nursing Practice. 2nd Ed., New York: J.B. Lippincott Co., 1978, pp. 441-453.

5. Falconer, M. et al.: The Drug-The Nurse-The Patient. 6th Ed., Philadelphia: W.B. Saunders Co., 1978, pp. 305-309, 323-330.

6. Friedman, H. H., (Ed.): Problem-Oriented Medical Diagnosis. Boston: Little, Brown and Co., 1975, pp. 54-64.

7. Guidelines for Educating Nurses in High Blood Pressure Control. DHEW Publication Number (N.I.H.) 77-1241.

8. Hartshorn, J.: What to Do When the Patient's in Hypertensive Crisis. Nursing 80 (July 1980): 36-45.

9. Hill, M.: Hypertension. What Can Go Wrong When You Measure Blood Pressure. Am J Nurs 80 (May 1980): 942-946.

10. Hussar, D.: New Drugs of 1978-79. Nursing 79 (May 1979): 32-40.

11. Sackett, D.: Hypertension III: The Hypertensive Workup. Can J Publ Health 71 (January/February 1980): 12-15.

12. Kannel, W. et al.: Role of Blood Pressure in the Development of Congestive Heart Failure. N Engl J Med 287 (October 19, 1972): 781-787.

13. Kaplan, N. M.: When Hypertension is Mild or Moderate. Drug Ther Vol. 5, No. 6 (June 1975): 43-47

14. Kirkendall, W.: When Hypertension is Malignant and Critical. Drug Ther Vol. 5, No. 6 (June 1975): 51-62

15. Laragh, J. H.: Hypertension. Drug Ther Hospital Edition Vol. 5 No. 1 (January 1980): 47-64.

16. Long, M. et al.: Hypertension: What Patients Need to Know. Am J Nurs 76 (May 1976): 765-769.

17. Luckmann, J. and Sorensen, K.: Medical-Surgical Nursing, A Psychophysiologic Approach. Philadelphia: W.B. Saunders Co., 1974, pp. 677-685, 1980, 863-878.

18. Marcinek, M. B.: Hypertension. What It Does To The Body. Am J Nurs 80 (May 1980): 928-932.

19. Merck Sharp & Dohme (compilers). The Hypertension Handbook. West Point, Pa., 1974, p. 76.

20. Moore, M.: Hypertensive Emergencies. Am Fam Physician 21 (March 1980): 141-146.

21. Moser, M.: Tips on Working Up Hypertensive Patients: When Have You Done Enough? Mod Med 48 (April 30, 1980): 24-32.

22. Moser, M.: Hypertension. How Therapy Works. Am J Nurs 80 (May 1980): 937-941.

23. Ross, A. et al.: Beta-Blockers: New Uses, New Benefits. Patient Care (December 15, 1979): 16-52.

24. Schoof, C.: Hypertension. Common Questions Patients Ask. Am J Nurs 80 (May 1980): 926-927.

25. Thind, G.: Factors Influencing Hypertension Prognosis and Treatment. Pract Cardiol 6 (April 1980): 31-38.

26. Veterans Administration Cooperative Study Group on Antihypertensive Agents: II. Results in Patients with Diastolic Blood Pressures Averaging 90 through 114 mm Hg. J Am Med Assoc 213 (August 1970): 1143-1152.

27. Wagner, E. H. et al.: Hypertension Control in a Rural Biracial Community: Successes and Failures of Primary Care. Am J Publ Health 70 (January 1980): 48-55.

28. White, S. and Williamson, K.: What to Watch For With Peripherally Acting Antihypertensives. RN (January 1980): 51-53.

29. Fink, J.W.: The Challenge of High Blood Pressure Control. Nurs C N Am 16 (June 1981): 301-308.

CHAPTER 16

MYOCARDIAL INFARCTION

LEARNING OBJECTIVES

Study of this chapter will enable the reader to:

1. Describe the myocardial changes that take place after a myocardial infarction (MI)

2. Differentiate between a type A and type B personality

3. Recognize symptoms which may indicate myocardial infarction

4. Describe initial objective data (signs) commonly found during the physical assessment of the client experiencing a myocardial infarction

5. Plan nursing interventions which support vital life processes, rest, and prevent complications

6. Discuss adaptive patterns which the client may display following MI

7. Assess the client's understanding of the alteration and how he/she expects it to change his/her lifestyle

8. Utilize community resources to facilitate the client's rehabilitative process

DESCRIPTION

Myocardial infarction (MI) is commonly referred to as a "heart attack." In myocardial infarction, an area of the myocardium (heart muscle) undergoes necrosis as a result of oxygen deprivation.[16] The oxygen deprivation is due to an obstruction or occlusion of one of the main coronary arteries (or their branches) which normally supplies the myocardium with blood. 16, 20

The left ventricle is one of the most common sites of myo-cardial infarction because this chamber has the greatest work load. 16

Necrosis of the infarcted area is evident within 5 to 6 hours after the occlusion. 16 The body's response to this necrosis is an increase in the production of leukocytes to aid in the removal of dead cells. The area of infarction is sur-rounded by an "area of injury," which is less severely damaged. The area of injury is bordered by the outermost area of damage referred to as the "zone of ischemia. "16 The area of injury and the zone of ischemia usually regain their function in 2 to 3 weeks after the onset of the occlusion. 16

The formation of a fibrous scar tissue usually is complete within 2 to 3 months. 16, 20 Myocardial infarction is the leading cause of death in the United States. 1

ETIOLOGY

Occlusion of a coronary blood vessel may be the result of:

1. Clot formation that develops suddenly, when an ather-omatous plaque ruptures through the sublayers of a blood vessel

2. When the roughened inner lining of a sclerosed artery leads to thrombosis 4, 16, 20

Myocardial infarction may also be the result of a sudden in-creased need for blood supply to the heart such as occurs in shock, hemorrhage, and severe physical exertion. 16 Aortic stenosis causes a restriction of blood flow through the aorta and predisposes one to the formation of emboli. 16

Cardiologists Friedman and Rosenman have engaged in re-search that has demonstrated that behavior patterns and certain types of modern day stress are among the principal culprits in the increased incidence of heart attacks among middle-aged Americans. 27 These cardiologists became convinced that people can be divided into two personality types:

1. Type A: the coronary-prone individual possessing
   traits such as: being aggressive, hard-driving, self-
   willed, intensely competitive, obsessively ambitious,
   constantly battling deadlines, always punctual, cannot
   stand to wait, has a harrowing sense of time urgency,
   has trouble facing self-insecurity and weakness, even
   though accomplishments are significant.

2. Type B: personality type is the converse of type A.[27]

   Professor Holmes (Department of Psychiatry) at the University of Washington has suggested that the "general rate of
change" in a person's life could be one of the most important
environmental factors leading to stress and ultimately myocardial infarction.[27] Professor Holmes and psychiatrist Richard
Rahe developed a research tool (The Life-Change Units Scale)
which assigns point values to changes. When yearly changes
add up to 300, according to the scale, a danger point has been
reached. They found that 80% of the clients who exceeded 300
became seriously depressed, had heart attacks or other serious
illnesses.[27]

   Hans Selye, M.D., the world's leading authority on
stress, defines diseases of adaptation as the consequences
of the body's inability to meet external agents by adequate
adaptive reaction.[27] Stress, in itself, is not always a harmful thing. It is the repeated exposure and reaction to continued or extreme stress that appear to cause illness, accident, and exhaustion (death).[27]

ASSESSMENT SPECIFIC TO THE ALTERATION

Subjective Data

   The most outstanding symptom may be a sudden sensation
of pressure or "crushing pain" in the chest.[16,31] This pain
may radiate to the arms, throat, and back, and may persist for
hours. Other client complaints may be: nausea and vomiting,
dyspnea, fatigue, faintness, or weakness.[9,31]

   Clients who have a highly developed collateral circulation
may suffer myocardial damage, but do not always experience
such vivid symptoms. These are sometimes referred to as
"silent coronaries."[1] Some clients may experience symptoms
of congestive heart failure and pulmonary edema (see Chapter
14 for these symptoms).

Objective Data

Initial signs of myocardial infarction occurring within the first 24 hours are:

1. General appearance of the client can vary considerably: he/she may be pale, diaphoretic, dyspneic, restless, apprehensive and clutching his/her chest or lies quietly, complains of pain, but may be sitting up trying to belch or even trying to walk to relieve the pain.

2. Vital signs: initially the blood pressure may be elevated, normal, or decreased; the heart rate is usually within normal limits (60 to 100 beats per minute); bradycardia (40 to 60 beats per minute) may be present, especially if it is an inferior wall infarction; sinus tachycardia (100 or more beats per minute) suggests that complications are likely to result; body temperature may be normal initially, but may be followed by a slight elevation; respiratory rate varies between 12 and 20 per minute, however, some clients experiencing pain or left heart failure may have tachypnea.

3. Premature ventricular contractions are common.

4. Arrhythmias may be present (see Chapter 12).

5. Cardiac examination

   a. Jugular venous pressure usually is not elevated initially.

   b. Pulmonary edema with rales and/or rhonchi bilaterally without increased jugular venous pressure may occur in the first few hours after infarction.

   c. Cardiac impulse usually is palpated in the normal position unless previous infarction, hypertension, or other causes of heart disease are present.

   d. Abnormal movements of the apical impulse may be palpated even though cardiomegaly is absent (a "bulge" may be felt).

e. Auscultation of heart sounds may be of normal intensity in most clients; phonocardiograms have demonstrated a reduction in intensity of both the first and the second sound after acute myocardial infarction; an audible atrial or fourth sound gallop has been observed in most clients. (It may be related to increased filling pressure in the left ventricle and temporary impairment of left ventricular function or decreased compliance of the left ventricle.)[24]

Electrocardiographic changes may appear within 24 hours after symptoms begin or they may be delayed as long as 5 to 6 days. Acute myocardial infarction is characterized by:

1. ST elevation (reflects myocardial ischemia)

2. T wave inversion (reflects the development of inflammation)

3. Q wave changes (indicate necrosis)[1]

It is important to remember that the ECG is considered along with the client's clinical status.

Laboratory findings that support the diagnosis of myocardial infarction are:

1. Leukocytosis and an elevated sedimentation rate reflect the inflammatory process.

2. Enzymes are released from the injured myocardial muscle: CPK, SGOT, and LDH become elevated after acute myocardial infarction.

Serum enzymes and other diagnostic tests are discussed in Chapter 4.

CLIENT CARE GOALS

Short-term goals:

1. Reduction of client's cardiac work load

2. Stabilize and maintain client's vital functions during the acute process

3. Relief of pain, dyspnea, and anxiety

4. Assist client in his/her adaptation to the cardiac alteration physically and psychologically

5. Educate client in regard to the disease process, cardiac risk factors, and prescribed medical regimen to prevent the recurrence of illness

Long-term goals:

Encourage the client to accept responsibility for his health care by complying with the prescribed medical regimen

Restore and maintain the client at his/her optimal level of functioning (physiologic, psychologic, and sociocultural)

INTERVENTIONS

Medical and nursing interventions are aimed at: supporting vital life processes, facilitating the healing process, and preventing complications.

Supportive Care

Initially, the client is admitted to a coronary care unit (CCU). It is generally accepted that coronary care units have been effective in reducing hospital mortality and that they offer the "optimum" in management of the client undergoing an acute myocardial infarction. [9] The client should be continuously monitored (ECG, vital signs, clinical signs and symptoms, etc.) in a CCU during the first 3 to 5 days of hospitalization.

An intravenous route should be established as soon as possible to administer emergency medications should the need arise.

Interventions are planned to facilitate the client's physical and mental rest. Rest reduces metabolic demands for oxygen and therefore reduces the workload of the heart. [1] Although on bed rest, most clients are allowed to use the bed side commode for bowel movements. [1,28] Some physicians allow their clients to rest sitting up in a special cardiac chair. Stool softeners are frequently ordered so that straining during defecation can be avoided. [1] Clients should be instructed to avoid the Valsalva maneuver (holding the breath and straining forces air against the closed glottis and raises the intrathoracic pressure interfering with venous return to the heart when the air is exhaled; the increased intrathoracic pressure falls and there is a sudden increase in venous return to the heart. [1] Activities that can precipitate a

Valsalva maneuver are: straining at stool, getting on and off the bedpan, pulling oneself up in bed, etc.[1]

Consideration should be given to the fact that, although bed rest is important, the client can experience many of the "hazards of immobility." Nursing and medical interventions should be planned to prevent these hazards (i.e., position changes, skin care, deep breathing, passive range of motion exercises, etc.). Sedatives are frequently prescribed to promote sleep. Relief of pain can be obtained by the use of morphine or meperidine.[28] A second dose of morphine should not be given if respirations are below 12 per minute.[28] The administration of oxygen is often useful for the relief of dyspnea, cyanosis, pulmonary edema, shock, and chest pain.

Ambulation and other activities are increased as the client's condition progresses satisfactorily.[1]

The client's psychologic needs must be met if "mental rest" is to be achieved. The client may be experiencing feelings of anxiety, fear of impending death, helplessness, dependency, inactivity, possible incapacity, insult to body image, and sexual inadequacy.[1] Adaptive patterns may include:

1. Phase I: shock and disbelief (approximately from 24 to 48 hours)-- behavioral responses may include anxiety, denial, or possibly aggressive sexual behavior.

2. Phase II: developing awareness (begins after 48 hours)-- reality sets in and the client's response may be one of depression and anger.

3. Phase III: resolution (begins after discharge)-- the client tries to deal with the consequences of myocardial infarction, gives up some of his dependence, and tries to assume responsibility for realistic goal-setting and planning interventions to achieve them; the client may experience all of the behavioral responses of the first two phases.[26]

Some nursing interventions to decrease the client's anxiety include:

1. Establishing a trusting nurse-client relationship

2. Orienting the client and family to the CCU

3. Explaining all procedures

4. Encouraging verbalization of questions, concerns, and feelings 26,31

The client's anxiety level is especially high:

On admission to the coronary care unit

Upon transfer from the coronary care unit

Prior to discharge[26]

by:
The nurse can sometimes deal with the client's depression

Letting him know that depression is a normal response when a person is hospitalized

Listening to the client express fears and feelings

Allowing the client to express anger without feeling guilty

If the client is extremely upset, the nurse should not try to reason with him at that time[26]

The client who feels that his masculinity is threatened may display aggressive sexual behavior toward the nurse. The nurse can intervene by being truthful with the client by:

Telling him that his behavior makes her uncomfortable

Asking the client if she has done something to stimulate his behavior

Accepting the client's behavior by realizing that his flirtatious compliments are attempts to bolster his ego[26]

Medication

The use of anticoagulant therapy (heparin and oral antico-agulants) in myocardial infarction continues to be a controversial matter. The three main purposes of anticoagulant therapy in acute MI (short-term therapy) are:

1. To prevent the development of venous thrombosis and

the risk of pulmonary embolism

2. To prevent the development of mural thrombi inside the heart and the risk of systemic embolization

3. To prevent appositional growth of the coronary thrombus in proximal direction with resulting extension of the MI [2, 6]

Long-term therapy with anticoagulants after a myocardial infarction is more controversial than short-term therapy. [2] The purposes given for long-term therapy include prevention of new coronary thrombosis and reinfarction. [2] Bjerkelund states that thromboembolic complications in the chronic stage of the disease are not frequent or serious enough to indicate long-term therapy. [2] Some physicians feel that all hospitalized clients with suspected or established acute MI should receive prophylactic anticoagulant therapy against the development of thromboembolic complications. [6] Sokolow states that anticoagulant therapy is usually recommended in severe cases of MI. [28] (Anticoagulants may be found in the Appendix.)

Vasodilator therapy (i.e., sodium nitroprusside, phentolamine, nitroglycerin) and diuretics have been utilized in the treatment of "pump failure" complicating a recent MI. [5, 28] Antiarrhythmic agents are discussed in the Appendix; digitalis preparations are discussed in Chapter 14.

Diet

The client's diet progresses from liquid to soft as tolerated. [1] Sodium restriction may or may not be prescribed. Controversy remains as to whether or not ice water should be restricted. Some authorities feel that ice water, hot drinks, and other stimulants can cause arrhythmias; others challenge this claim. [1] Obese clients may be placed on a weight reduction diet.

Education

Client education continues to be extremely important. The teaching content should be defined and the information presented by various health team members should be coordinated, so that excessive repetition and contradictory information is avoided. [32] Suggested instructional content includes:

Discussion of the disease process

Review the means of reducing coronary risk factors

Physical activity

Sexual activity

Dietary alterations

Importance of scheduled rest periods

Medical follow-up and adhering to the medical regimen

Signs and symptoms requiring medical assistance

Daily weights

Information regarding prescribed medications (name, action, dosage, route of administration, side effects, and toxicity)[1]

The client should be informed of the community resources available to facilitate the rehabilitative process: public health nurse, American Heart Association, and coronary clubs.[1] Some communities have active rehabilitation programs whose goal is to improve and restore cardiovascular function through progressive exercise under medical supervision.

COMPLICATIONS

Cardiac failure, cardiogenic shock, arrhythmias, Stokes-Adams attack with heart block, thromboembolic phenomena, oliguria, anuria, acute tubular necrosis, cardiac rupture, perforation of the interventricular septum, mitral insufficiency from papillary dysfunction or rupture, and ventricular aneurysm are all possible complications.[28]

REVIEW QUESTIONS

1. After myocardial infarction the myocardium undergoes changes. Describe these changes.

2. What is the body's response to myocardial necrosis?

3. How long does it usually take for the formation of a fibrous

scar to develop over the infarcted myocardial area?

4. What is the etiology of myocardial infarction?

5. Describe the characteristic traits of a person with a type A personality.

6. Does stress play a role in the development of a myocardial infarction? Explain your answer.

7. Is stress always harmful to a person?

8. What is the outstanding symptom in myocardial infarction?

9. Although the appearance of the client experiencing a myocardial infarction can vary considerably, what are some frequent general signs?

10. Name the three enzymes that become elevated after an acute myocardial infarction.

11. What is the rationale behind interventions to promote rest in the client experiencing a myocardial infarction?

12. Explain the Valsalva maneuver.

13. Identify at least four nursing interventions that could be implemented to prevent the "hazards of immobility."

14. Should morphine be administered to clients whose respirations are below 12 per minute?

15. Depression is not uncommon in postmyocardial infarction clients. Name at least five ways the nurse can deal with the client's depression.

16. In what ways could the nurse deal with a client of the opposite sex who is displaying aggressive sexual behavior?

17. List the three main purposes of anticoagulant therapy in acute myocardial infarction.

18. Client education continues to be a very important responsibility of the nurse. List topics that should be included in the instructional process.

19. Name three community resources available to facilitate the client's rehabilitative process.

20. What are some of the complications that may occur post-MI?

REFERENCES

1. Beyers, M. and Dudas, S.: The Clinical Practice of Medical-Surgical Nursing. Boston: Little, Brown and Co., 1977, pp. 347-368.

2. Bjerkelund, C.: Anticoagulant Therapy in Myocardial Infarction. Heart Lung 4 (January-February 1975): 61-68.

3. Cassem, N.H. and Hackett, T. P.: Psychological Rehabilitation of Myocardial Infarction Patients in the Acute Phase. Heart Lung 2 (May-June 1973): 382-388.

4. Chandler, A.: Relationship of Coronary Thrombosis to M.I. Mod Conc Cardiovasc Dis 44 (January 1975): 1-6.

5. Chatterjee, K. and Swan, H. J. C.: Vasodilator Therapy in Acute M.I. Mod Conc Cardiovasc Dis 43 (November 1974): 119-124.

6. Copans, H. and Lakier, J.: Commonly Encountered Problems in Anticoagulant Therapy. Pract Cardiol 6 (July 1980): 23-31.

7. Crawshaw, J.: Community Rehabilitation After Acute Myocardial Infarction. Heart Lung 3 (March-April 1974): 258-262.

8. Denzler, T. et al.: Angina Pectoris and Myocardial Infarction in the Presence of Patent Coronary Arteries--A Review. Heart Lung 3 (July-August 1974): 646-653.

9. Duncan, B. and Fulton, M.: Events Surrounding an Acute Heart Attack. Community Aspects of Unstable Angina and the Acute Heart Attack. Heart Lung 4 (January-February 1975): 50-56.

10. Foster, S. B. et al.: Pump Failure Following Myocardial Infarction: An Overview. Heart Lung 9 (March-April 1980): 293-298.

11. Gentry, W. D.: Emotional and Behavioral Reaction to Acute M. I. Heart Lung 4 (September-October 1975): 738-745.

12. Harding, A. L. and Morefield, M. A.: Group Intervention for Wives of Myocardial Infarction Patients. Nurs Clin N Am 11 (June 1976): 338-346.

13. Johnston, B. et al.: Eight Steps to Inpatient Cardiac Rehabilitation: The Team Effort-Methodology and Preliminary Results. Heart Lung 5 (January-February 1976): 97-111.

14. Luchi, R. J. et al.: Use of Cardioactive Drugs in Acute Myocardial Infarction. Heart Lung 5 (January-February 1976): 44-61.

15. Mc Lane, M. et al.: Psychosexual Adjustment and Counseling After Myocardial Infarction. Ann Intern Med 92 (April 1980): 514-519.

16. Miller, B. and Keane, C.: Encyclopedia and Dictionary of Medicine, Nursing and Allied Health. 2nd Ed., Philadelphia: W. B. Saunders Co., 1978, pp. 663-664.

17. Moskowitz, L.: Vasodilator Therapy in Acute Myocardial Infarction. Heart Lung 4 (November-December 1975): 939-945.

18. Mullins, C. B. and Atkins, J.: Prognoses and Management of Ventricular Conduction Blocks in Acute Myocardial Infarction. Mod Conc Cardiovasc Dis 45 (October 1976): 129-134.

19. Norris, R. M.: Prognosis in Myocardial Infarction. Heart Lung 4 (January-February 1975): 75-80.

20. Oliver, M. F.: The Metabolic Response to a Heart Attack. Heart Lung 4 (January-February 1975): 57-60.

21. O'Rourke, M.: Cardiogenic Shock Following M. I. Heart Lung 3 (March-April 1974): 252-257.

22. Pole, D.: Delays Between Onset of Acute M. I. and Definitive Care. Heart Lung 3 (March-April 1974): 263-267.

23. Rahe, R. H. et al.: A Teaching Evaluation Questionnaire for Postmyocardial Infarction Patients. Heart Lung 4 (September-October 1975): 759-766.

24. Romhilt, D. and Fowler, N.: Physical Signs in Acute Myocardial Infarction. Heart Lung 2 (January-February 1973): 74-80.

25. Sawaya, M. et al.: Hemorrhagic Cardiac Tamponade Complicating the Postmyocardial Infarction Syndrome in the Absence of Anticoagulation. Heart Lung 4 (September-October 1975): 770-774.

26. Scalzi, C.: Nursing Management of Behavioral Responses Following an Acute Myocardial Infarction. Heart Lung 2 (January-February 1973): 62-69

27. Slay, C. L.: Myocardial Infarction and Stress. Nurs Clin N Am 11 (June 1976): 329-338.

28. Sokolow, M.: Heart and Great Vessels. In Krupp, M.A. and Chatton, M.J.: Current Medical Diagnosis and Treatment. Los Altos, Calif.: Lange Medical Publications, 1976, pp. 193-201.

29. Thompson, D. R.: Resuscitation of Patients With Cardiac Arrest Following Myocardial Infarction. Nurs Times 76 (January 3, 1980): 36-37.

30. Collins, J. and Brigham, P.: Understanding Anticoagulation Therapy. Patient Care 13 (November 15, 1979): 76-78.

31. Webb, K. A,: A Patient With Myocardial Infarction. Nurs Times 76 (January 1980): 74-77.

32. Wenger, N. and Mount, F.: An Educational Algorithm Myocardial Infarction. Cardiovasc Nurs 10 (May-June 1974): 11-16

33. Yan, V.: Pericarditis in Acute Myocardial Infarction. Heart Lung 3 (March-April 1974): 247-251.

CHAPTER 17

PULMONARY EMBOLISM

LEARNING OBJECTIVES

Study of this chapter will enable the reader to:

1. Discuss factors which promote thrombus formation

2. Identify clients who are at risk for the development of pulmonary embolism

3. Describe diagnostic tests available to confirm the diagnosis of pulmonary embolism

4. Plan nursing interventions aimed at the prevention of deep venous thrombosis

5. Assess high-risk clients at frequent intervals in order to ensure earlier recognition of the occurrence of pulmonary embolism

6. Design a teaching plan to assist the client in understanding the potential complications associated with the use of anticoagulants and the signs and symptoms that should be reported immediately to the physician

7. Evaluate the effectiveness of client care given by the health team members in relation to established goals

DESCRIPTION

Pulmonary embolism is characterized by sudden, acute respiratory distress (i.e., tachypnea, restlessness, dyspnea, and pleural pain).[1] It is not an infrequent complication of medical or surgical care. Some authorities state that pulmonary embolism is the most frequently encountered pulmonary illness in a general hospital.[7] Pulmonary emboli frequently arise from thrombi in the deep veins of the lower limbs, where the thrombi become detached and are carried to the lungs. [7]

Factors which have been proposed as promoting the formation of thrombi are:

1. Stasis of blood

2. Vessel wall changes

3. Hypercoagulability of blood. [7]

Dislodgment or fragmentation of thrombi may be due to:

1. Mechanical forces: direct trauma, sudden muscle action, or changes in blood flow rate which may cause unusual intravascular pressure changes

2. Spontaneous fragmentation: caused by the natural mechanism of clot dissolution [7]

High-risk groups include clients experiencing:

1. Cardiac disease (especially congestive heart failure)

2. Chronic lung disease

3. Thrombophlebitis

4. Recent surgery

5. A fractured hip

6. Malignancy

7. Previous pulmonary embolism [7]

ETIOLOGY

Factors promoting thrombus formation have already been presented in the description of pulmonary embolism. The etiology of pulmonary embolism may be a combination of factors such as:

1. The advancing age of the client coming to surgery

2. Increasing the duration of bed rest

3. Possible deterioration of the client's nutritional state [7]

It is estimated that more than 85% of pulmonary emboli arise from the deep venous system of the lower extremities; the remaining few arise from the pelvic veins or right atrium. [8]

ASSESSMENT SPECIFIC TO THE ALTERATION

Signs and symptoms will vary from mild to severe depending on the extent of lung involvement.

Subjective Data

The client's symptoms are often nonspecific and may be overlooked.

Nonspecific symptoms may include:

1. Dyspnea (the client may complain of not being able to take a deep breath)

2. Cough (usually nonproductive and annoying)

3. Pleural pain

4. Hemoptysis (blood-streaked sputum rather than frank bleeding) [7]

Objective Data

Physical signs are equally nonspecific:

1. Accentuated pulmonary second sound (P2)

2. Tachypnea (more than 20 respirations per minute)

3. Rales

4. Tachycardia (more than 100 beats per minute)

5. Mild temperature elevation

6. Gallop rhythm

7. Chest splinting

8. Cyanosis

Laboratory tests are also nonspecific for pulmonary embolism:

1. WBC may range from less than 10, 000 to below 15, 000

2. There is no characteristic serum enzyme pattern (LDH, SGOT)

3. Elevation in serum bilirubin often correlates with the presence of right heart failure rather than pulmonary embolism [7]

Arterial blood gas studies are useful in establishing a diagnosis if the client does not have preexisting cardiopulmonary disease. If the Pao2 is above 90 mm Hg, the diagnosis of pulmonary embolism is unlikely. [7] Although the ECG is not a very sensitive or specific diagnostic tool for pulmonary embolism, some clients develop changes such as sudden atrial fibrillation or flutter, other supraventricular tachycardias, and ventricular ectopic beats. [7] Dr. L. Berman and others have stated that acute pulmonary embolism is always associated with a sinus or other supraventricular tachyarrhythmia and that the strain on the right ventricle is evidenced by:

1. Elevated ST segments and inverted T waves most marked in the right precordial leads

2. Wide frontal plane QRS-T angle with the T wave axis deviated to the left and incomplete right bundle branch block which reflects right ventricular diastolic overload [2]

The routine chest x-ray is often nonspecific if infarction has not occurred. [10]
Some common findings are:

A high diaphragm on the embolized side

Pleural fluid

Plump pulmonary arteries

Sudden cutoff of a pulmonary artery shadow

Decreased vascular markings

A small bilateral or large unilateral effusion [7]

A normal chest x-ray would not be unusual. Radioisotope lung scanning, although it is a nonspecific test, is the procedure of choice in screening clients for pulmonary emboli.[7] The test itself can only be interpreted as normal or abnormal. There will be radioactivity wherever blood flow exists in the lung.[7, 10] If emboli are present, the amount of radioactive substance will be decreased or absent. It must be remembered that conditions other than pulmonary emboli will alter blood flow to the lungs. These conditions include: congestive heart failure, pneumonia, tumor, chronic lung disease, etc. When other diseases are present, pulmonary angiography may be needed to confirm the diagnosis of pulmonary emboli. This procedure is more complex than radioisotope scanning, in that a radiopaque contrast material is injected under pressure by a catheter inserted into the pulmonary artery.[7] The site of the obstruction and the clot can be visually detected.[7, 10]

CLIENT CARE GOALS

1. Prevention of thromboembolic complications

2. Early recognition of pulmonary embolism

3. Implementation of interventions to promote the resolution of thromboembolic complications and prevent their recurrence

4. Provide for client education and discharge planning

INTERVENTIONS

Nursing and medical interventions aimed at the prevention of deep venous thrombosis are of utmost importance. Precisely because of the subtle and nonspecific signs and symptoms of pulmonary embolism, all health team members should make astute observations of changes in the client's condition. Increases in temperature, heart rate, respiratory rate, and complaints of dyspnea should be carefully evaluated by the nurse and brought to the attention of the physician. Nurses should use their assessment skills and clinical knowledge to assess high-risk clients frequently, so that "earlier recognition" of pulmonary emboli is realized. Since the nurse is frequently, held responsible for client education, the nurse has an opportunity to instruct the hospitalized client on how venous thrombosis can be prevented.

Client instruction should include:

1. Active and passive leg exercises to increase venous return

2. Elevation of extremities

3. Use of elastic stockings

4. The importance of early ambulation

5. Quadriceps contractions

6. The dangers of prolonged sitting and leg crossing

7. Avoidance of wearing constrictive garments 8

Female clients who have experienced embolism should not take oral contraceptives. 4 Some physicians are using low-weight dextran on their hospitalized clients to prevent deep venous thrombosis. 8

During the acute phase of pulmonary embolism, heparin is the anticoagulant of choice. Heparin can be administered by:

1. Intermittent IV infusion mixed in a small amount of fluid (piggy-back set-up)

2. Intermittent injection into a heparin lock (heparin bolus)

3. Continuous infusion

4. Deep subcutaneous injection (injection sites should be rotated systematically and inspected carefully before and after injections for the presence of hematomas) 7

Surgical interruption of the inferior vena cava may be performed such as: ligation, clipping, plication, and filter. Other procedures include: the intracaval umbrella filter (performed under local anesthesia), pulmonary embolectomy, and thrombolytic therapy with agents such as streptokinase or urokinase. 7 Oral anticoagulants are frequently prescribed during the chronic phase of pulmonary embolism. Clients being discharged on oral anticoagulants must understand the potential complications associated with the use of anticoagulants.

Signs and symptoms that the client should look for and report immediately include:

Epistaxis

Petechiae

Bleeding gums

Ecchymosis

Dark red or coffee-
colored urine [6]

Hematomas

Tarry stools

Clients should be warned not to take aspirin or any salicylate drug without specific orders from their physician, since they tend to depress blood clotting.

Oral anticoagulants have a great number of interactions with other drugs and are enhanced by:

Phenylbutazone

Anabolic agents

Sulfonamides

Quinidine

Clofibrate

Salicylates

D-Thyroxine

Bromelains (anti-inflammatory
agents)

Papain (a proteolytic
enzyme) [6]

Oral anticoagulants are inhibited by: sedatives, haloper-
idol (antipsychotic drug), griseofulvin. [6]

COMPLICATIONS

Massive pulmonary embolism can result in death within minutes. [8] The clinical picture tends more toward sudden, pro-
found shock with sympathetic overactivity, cyanosis, tachypnea with mental clouding, or anxiety. [3] In a massive embolus, when anorexia and shock are established, ventricular arrhythmias may emerge. [3]

Complications of Pulmonary Angiography

Arrhythmias can occur while the catheter transverses the right ventricle into the pulmonary artery. [10] Other local complications include: infection at the cutdown site of the arm,

formation of a hematoma in the groin when a percutaneous transfemoral venous approach is used.[10] Anaphylactic reaction to the contrast media is possible. Perforation of the cardiac wall by the catheter can result in hemorrhage into the pericardium and pericardial tamponade.[10]

REVIEW QUESTIONS

1. List three factors which promote thrombus formation.

2. Name seven groups of clients who are at high risk for pulmonary embolism.

3. The etiology of pulmonary emboli may be a combination of factors. Name at least three of these factors.

4. From what system do 85% of pulmonary emboli arise?

5. Name four nonspecific symptoms which may be overlooked in the client experiencing a pulmonary embolism.

6. Which diagnostic test is the procedure of choice in screening clients for pulmonary emboli?

7. Heparin is the anticoagulant of choice in the acute phase of pulmonary embolism. By what four methods can heparin be administered?

8. Oral anticoagulants may cause complications. What signs and symptoms should the client look for and report immediately?

9. Name several complications of pulmonary embolism.

10. What complications are possible when pulmonary angiography is performed?

REFERENCES

1. Baldwin, L.: The Problem of Pulmonary Embolism. Heart Lung 3 (March-April 1974): 207-208.

2. Berman, L. and Schamroth, L.: Acute Pulmonary Embolism. Heart Lung 8 (November-December 1979): 1146-1147.

214/ Part III

3. Bloomfield, D. A.: The Recognition and Management of Massive Pulmonary Embolism. Heart Lung 3 (March-April 1974): 241-246.

4. Brunner, L. and Suddarth, D.: The Lippincott Manual of Nursing Practice. 2nd Ed., New York: J.B. Lippincott Co., 1978, p. 261.

5. Daly, C. R. and Kelly, E. A.: Prevention of Pulmonary Embolism: Intra-Caval Devices. Am J Nurs 72 (1972): 2004.

6. Falconer, M. et al.: The Drug-The Nurse-The Patient. 6th Ed., Philadelphia: W.B. Saunders Co., 1978, pp. 317-320.

7. Fitzmaurice, J. and Sasahara, A.: Current Concepts of Pulmonary Embolism: Implications for Nursing Practice. Heart Lung 3 (March-April 1974): 209-218.

8. Genton, E.: Therapeutic Aspects of Pulmonary Embolism. Heart Lung 3 (March-April 1974): 233-236.

9. Gray, F. D.: Pulmonary Embolism: Avoiding the Diagnostic Pitfalls. Consultant 19 (April 1979): 71-72.

10. Grollman, J.: Radiological Diagnosis of Pulmonary Thromboembolism. Heart Lung 3 (March-April 1974): 219-226

11. Perlman, M. M.: Electrocardiographic Changes in Acute Pulmonary Embolism. Heart Lung 1 (November-December 1972): 831-834.

12. Wilson, A. et al.: Radioisotopic Diagnosis of Pulmonary Embolism. Heart Lung 3 (March-April 1974): 227-232.

CHAPTER 18

RAYNAUD DISEASE

LEARNING OBJECTIVES

Study of this chapter will enable the reader to:

1. Describe the common characteristics of Raynaud disease

2. Discuss precipitating factors in relation to Raynaud disease

3. Identify sensory changes which may be found in the client experiencing Raynaud disease

4. Develop a teaching care plan to assist the client in identification and elimination of precipitating factors

5. Recommend relaxation techniques if emotional stress is identified as a precipitating factor

6. Evaluate interventions for their effectiveness in alleviating the client's discomfort

DESCRIPTION

Raynaud disease tends to occur primarily in young females who are between puberty and 40 years of age. [5] The disease is characterized by intermittent attacks of bilateral, symmetrical pallor and cyanosis followed by rubor of the skin of the fingers (rarely in the toes); gangrene may be absent or minimal near the fingertips. [4, 5] Ischemia usually starts in the fingertips and progresses proximally. [7]

Attacks may be precipitated by exposure to cold or by emotional upsets and are relieved by warmth. [5, 7] Some authors report that there is a hereditary tendency in about one-half of the clients. [1, 5, 6]

ETIOLOGY

Unknown. It is thought to be due to an abnormality of the
sympathetic nervous system. [5], [7]

ASSESSMENT SPECIFIC TO THE ALTERATION

Signs and symptoms of Raynaud disease are the result of
excessive vasoconstriction and digital ischemia which predominantly involves the hands. [2]

Subjective Data

The client's history reveals a long period of sensitivity to
cold.

The following events occur on exposure to cold:

1. The client's fingers (occasionally the toes) become
blanched and white in appearance and numb (due to
vasospasm).

2. Later the whiteness and pallor changes to cyanosis
(due to retarded flow of poorly oxygenated blood in the
capillaries and venules).

3. When the vasospasm terminates, circulation is restored to the affected digits, reactive hyperemia
(rubor) occurs, and is followed by a return of normal
color to the digits. [2], [5], [7]

The client also complains of an aching type of pain during the
attack. The thumbs are rarely affected. Each episode may
last from 15 to 60 minutes. [4]

Objective Data

Sensory changes may be found such as numbness, stiffness,
and diminished sensation. [5]

The disease is usually progressive and atrophy of the
terminal fat pads and the digital skin may be observed; gan-
grenous ulcers may occur near the fingertips. [4], [5]

Diagnosis usually is based on the long history of signs and
symptoms of Raynaud disease.

Laboratory findings are usually negative (CBC, ESR, anti-nuclear antibody, cryoglobulins, serum protein electrophoresis (SPEP), urinalysis).[7] Other diseases should be ruled out such as: thromboangitis obliterans, arteriosclerosis obliterans, thoracic outlet syndrome, collagen diseases, and cryoglobulinemia.[5]

CLIENT CARE GOAL

Vasospasm will be prevented or relieved through the identification and elimination of precipitating factors.

INTERVENTIONS

The health team member should encourage the client to give up smoking, if this is a probable precipitating factor. The client should be assisted in identifying causative factors which may be provoking spasm (i.e., exposure to cold, emotional upsets, drugs, toxins, etc.)[3]

Agents reported to have caused digital ischemia include: ergot compounds, methysergide, beta-adrenergic blockers, sympathomimetic drugs, and oral contraceptives. [7]

Once causative factors have been identified, a plan should be developed to avoid these factors. Vasodilators may be prescribed (e.g., phenoxybenzamine, (Dibenzyline), cyclandelate, (Cyclospasmol), or tolazoline (Priscoline).[3] Agents that may decrease peripheral vasoconstriction have been used in selected cases (reserpine, prazosin).[7] If the preceding conservative methods are ineffective, a regional sympathectomy, which would remove vasoconstricting impulses, may be considered.[3]

It has been found that early after sympathectomy, the digital blood flow is increased; after several weeks, the flow returns to preoperative rates. [7] Many physicians feel that sympathectomy is inadequate in the treatment of Raynaud disease.

Although rare, amputation occasionally may be necessary when gangrene affects the digits.[3] When possible, the client may be advised to move to a warmer climate.

COMPLICATIONS

Complications are gangrene and possible amputation.

REVIEW QUESTIONS

1. Describe the characteristics of Raynaud disease.

2. Name two factors that may precipitate the attacks.

3. What sensory changes are found in Raynaud disease?

4. Raynaud disease may be treated by conservative methods such as?

5. If conservative methods are not effective, what other interventions are possible?

6. Name two complications of Raynaud disease.

REFERENCES

1. Armington, Sr. C. and Creighton, H.: Nursing of People with Cardiovascular Problems. Boston: Little, Brown and Co., 1971, pp. 261-262.

2. Beyers, M. and Dudas, S.: The Clinical Practice of Medical-Surgical Nursing. Boston: Little, Brown and Co., 1977, pp. 403-404.

3. Brunner, L. and Suddarth, D.: The Lippincott Manual of Nursing Practice. 2nd Ed., New York: J. B. Lippincott Co., 1978, pp. 440-441.

4. De Gowin, E. and De Gowin, R.: Bedside Diagnostic Evaluation. 2nd Ed., New York: Macmillan Co., 1969, pp. 413-414.

5. Erskine, J.: Blood Vessels and Lymphatics. In Krupp, M. A. and Chatton, M. J.: Current Medical Diagnosis and Treatment. Los Altos, Calif.: Lange Medical Publications, 1976, pp. 259-260.

6. Halperin, J. L.: Pathophysiology of Raynaud's Disease. Arch Intern Med (January 1979): 89.

7. Hoffman, G.: Raynaud's Disease and Phenomenon. Vol. 21, No. 1 Am Fam Physician (January 1980): 91-97.

8. Metzler, M. and Silver, D.: Vasospastic Disorders. Postgrad Med 66 (February 1979): 79.

9. Shafer, K. et al.: Medical-Surgical Nursing. 6th Ed., St. Louis: C. V. Mosby Co., 1975, pp. 387-388.

CHAPTER 19

RHEUMATIC HEART DISEASE

LEARNING OBJECTIVES

Study of this chapter will enable the reader to:

1. Discuss the cardiac complications possible after an episode of rheumatic fever

2. Describe the major and minor features of rheumatic fever

3. Discuss subjective and objective data in relation to mitral stenosis and/or aortic stenosis

4. Develop a plan of care for the client experiencing rheumatic fever

5. Describe commonly prescribed medical interventions and their rationale for the client experiencing rheumatic fever, mitral stenosis, and aortic stenosis

6. Employ preventative measures in the community to reduce the initial occurrence of rheumatic fever

7. Evaluate the effectiveness of client care and recommend alternatives as appropriate

DESCRIPTION

Rheumatic heart disease (RHD) occurs after one or more attacks of rheumatic fever. Endocarditis (inflammation of the inner lining of the heart and valve membranes) is a usual complication of rheumatic fever. [5] As healing occurs, the valves of the heart become scarred and stiff and are unable to close properly. This allows leakage of blood through the incompetent valve producing the characteristic heart murmur. If valve scarring becomes very thick, blood flow through the heart becomes restricted.

Rheumatic fever usually follows a group A beta-hemolytic streptococcal infection.[3] This febrile illness is seen most frequently in children between the ages of 5 and 10 years. An attack of rheumatic fever does not result in immunity; recurrences are possible.[6] The mitral valve is affected in 50 to 60% of the cases of rheumatic heart disease, 20% of the cases have combined lesions of the aortic and mitral valves, and 10% have pure aortic lesions.[7]

ETIOLOGY

RHD occurs as a complication of rheumatic fever. Some authorities feel that rheumatic fever develops as a hypersensitivity reaction to certain allergens; most evidence points to the theory of poststreptococcal hypersensitization.[4]

ASSESSMENT SPECIFIC TO THE ALTERATION

It is possible for rheumatic fever and RHD to go undiagnosed if the symptoms are mild or if no noticeable symptoms occur. RHD may be discovered years later.[6]

Subjective Data and Objective Data in Relation to Rheumatic Fever

The major clinical features include:

1. Polyarthritis: migratory involvement of the large joints of the body; the knees especially become tender, warm, reddened, and swollen

2. Carditis: may involve the myocardium, endocardium, or pericardium or all three layers may be involved simultaneously

3. Chorea: manifested by involuntary spasmodic movements of the extremities, incoordination, slurred speech, and facial grimacing

4. Nodules: hard, painless, nonpruritic swellings over the elbows, knuckles, knees, dorsum of the feet, and prominences of the dorsal spine

5. Erythema marginatum: a rash characterized by pink, nonpruritic, slightly raised macules with a distinct, wavy margin [3, 4]

Minor clinical manifestations include:

1. Fever

2. Arthralgia (joint pain without visible signs of inflamma-
    tion)

3. Epistaxis

4. Abdominal pain

5. ECG changes (atrioventricular conduction delay)

6. Elevated erythrocyte sedimentation test and C-react-
    ive protein

7. Past history of acute rheumatic fever [3]

Approximately 85 to 90% of the clients with rheumatic fever
have an elevation of the antistreptolysin serum titers, indicating
that the client's body has formed antibodies against one or
more streptococcal antigens. [4] The throat culture is positive
for beta-hemolytic group A streptococci in about 50% of the
clients with active rheumatic fever. [4]

Subjective and Objective Data in Relation to Mitral Stenosis

In mild cases, the client may be asymptomatic. In moderate stenosis, the client experiences dyspnea and fatigue on
exertion as the left atrial pressure rises. [7]

Clients with severe mitral stenosis have a high left atrial
pressure at rest which produces pulmonary venous congestion
at rest and worsens with exercise. [7] When the client reclines
for the night, the pulmonary blood volume increases causing:

1. Orthopnea

2. Paroxysmal nocturnal dyspnea

3. Actual transudation of fluid into the alveoli resulting
    in acute pulmonary edema and hemoptysis [6, 7]

Murmurs are sharply localized near the apex.

Special diagnostic tests that have proved helpful include:

Echocardiography

Left ventricular angiocardiography

Dye dilution

Pressure curves from the left ventricle and left atrium during left heart catheterization [7]

Subjective and Objective Data in Relation to Aortic Stenosis

The valve cusps become stiff and calcified and obstruct the blood flow resulting in an elevated left ventricular pressure and low cardiac output. Clinical symptoms may be few, but some clients experience fatigue, faintness, and angina. [6]

The chest x-ray may reveal a heart of normal size or with a slight enlargment of the left ventricle. [6]

Untreated aortic stenosis can result in congestive heart failure.

Murmurs may be heard in the second right intercostal space parasternally and/or near the apex. [7]

CLIENT CARE GOALS

1. Rheumatic heart disease will be prevented by preventing the occurence of its percursor, rheumatic fever.

2. Rheumatic fever will be prevented by controlling and alleviating group A hemolytic streptococcal infection.

3. The heart will be protected against the damaging effects of carditis.

4. Interventions will be implemented to relieve joint pain, fever, and other synptoms. [4,6]

INTERVENTIONS FOR THE CLIENT WITH RHEUMATIC FEVER

General

General interventions to care for the client with rheumatic fever include:

1. Bed rest to reduce the cardiac work load and metabolic needs during the acute stage.

2. Proper body alignment and protective handling of body joints.

3. Proper diet: a bland, high-protein, high-carbohydrate diet to maintain adequate nutrition while the client is experiencing fever and infection.

4. Drug therapy such as salicylates, antibiotics, and in some cases steroids (this is a controversial subject at this time). [1,4]

Medications

Salicylates are used primarily for their action of analgesia and antipyresis. Sodium bicarbonate should not be given with salicylates because it accelerates the excretion of salicylates and therefore reduces the efficiency of their absorption.

Early signs of salicylate toxicity include: tinnitus, nausea, and vomiting. [4] Less common side effects of salicylates include: headache, confusion, excessive perspiration, thirst, vomiting, skin rash, lassitude, and apathy.

Salicylate interactions:

1. They potentiate the action of penicillin, methotrexate, sulfonylurea, and para-aminosalicylic acid.

2. They counteract the uricosuric effect of probenecid and sulfinpyrazone.

3. Salicylates are enhanced by phenobarbital.

4. Salicylates should not be used concurrently with oral anticoagulants due to the additive effect seen when they are given at the same time.

Ideally, interventions should be aimed at prevention of rheumatic fever. The nurse often comes in contact with people in the community and should encourage prompt medical attention for children, teenagers, and young adults who have sore throats. [4] Prophylactic doses of antibiotics and good health practices can prevent subsequent attacks of rheumatic fever.

Complications

Serious complications of rheumatic fever include: congestive heart failure, infarctions of the brain or kidneys by emboli from valvular lesions or mural thrombi, bacterial endocarditis, and pulmonary congestion due to left-sided heart failure. [4]

INTERVENTIONS FOR MITRAL STENOSIS

Treatment of mitral stenosis may be:

1. Conservative: limitation of activity, sodium restriction, diuretics, and digitalis.

2. Surgical intervention called "mitral commissurotomy" to break apart the stenosed leaves of the mitral valve; a closed technique may be used. [6] If the closed technique is unsuccessful, open-heart surgery may be needed to replace the calcified valve with an artificial ball valve. Postoperative care is similar to that of other clients undergoing cardiac surgery.

INTERVENTIONS FOR AORTIC STENOSIS

Surgical intervention requires the use of extracorporeal circulation. Three methods may be used to repair the aortic valve:

1. Removal of calcium and opening of the fused commissures.

2. Reconstructing the aortic valve by removing one cusp.

3. The valve may be totally removed and replaced with artificial cusps or ball valves similar to those used for mitral valve replacement. [6]

Postoperative care is similar to that of other clients who have undergone cardiac surgery.

COMPLICATIONS

Complications have been included under subjective and objective data for each condition discussed.

REVIEW QUESTIONS

1. Does one attack of rheumatic fever result in immunity?

2. What is the etiology of rheumatic heart disease (RHD)?

3. Name five major clinical features of rheumatic fever (RF).

4. Name seven minor clinical features of RF.

5. List some general interventions to care for the client with RF.

6. When would be the best time to administer salicylates to prevent or minimize gastric distress?

7. Name three early signs of salicylate toxicity.

8. Salicylates should not be used concurrently with oral anticoagulants. What is the reason for this?

9. Serious complications from RF are possible. Name four.

10. What are three methods that can be used to repair the aortic valve which is stenosed?

11. How is mitral stenosis treated?

REFERENCES

1. Anthony, C.: Pediatric Cardiology. Garden City, NY: Medical Examination Publishing Co., Inc., 1979, pp. 438-448.

2. Coulehan, J. et al.: Acute Rheumatic Fever and Rheumatic Heart Disease on the Navajo Reservation, 1962-77. Pub Health Rep 95 (January-February 1980): 62-68.

3. Doyle, E.: Rheumatic Fever--A Continuing Problem. Cardovasc Nurs 10 (July-August 1974): 17-22.

4. Luckmann, J. and Sorensen, K.: Medical-Surgical Nursing, A Psychophysiological Approach. Philadelphia: W. B. Saunders Co., 1974, pp. 686-689, 1980, 879-883.

5. Miller, B. and Keane, C.: Encyclopedia and Dictionary of Medicine, Nursing and Allied Health. 2nd Ed., Philadelphia: W. B. Saunders Co., 1978, pp. 882-883.

6. Shafer, K. et al.: Medical-Surgical Nursing. 6th Ed., St. Louis: C. V. Mosby Co., 1975, pp. 332-335.

7. Sokolow, M.: Heart and Great Vessels. In Krupp, M. A. and Chatton, M. J.: Current Medical Diagnosis and Treatment. Los Altos, Calif.: Lange Medical Publications, 1976, pp. 165-174.

CHAPTER 20

SHOCK

LEARNING OBJECTIVES

Study of this chapter will enable the reader to:

1. Describe the four classifications of shock presented in this chapter

2. Demonstrate the ability to perform a rapid physical assessment of the client in a crisis situation

3. Collect and evaluate initial laboratory data

4. Detect the classic signs of shock

5. Select emergency interventions to promote tissue perfusion in the client experiencing shock

6. Evaluate the effectiveness of prescribed therapies in improving the client's physical and emotional status

7. Formulate and implement nursing interventions to prevent the occurrence of shock in all clients cared for

DESCRIPTION

Shock can be defined as a pathophysiologic state characterized by inadequate tissue perfusion which leads to generalized cellular hypoxia and vital organ damage. [5, 8] A drop in systolic blood pressure usually accompanies shock, but a normal blood pressure does not rule it out. Shock may be classified as:

Hypovolemic Shock

In hypovolemic shock the circulating blood volume is decreased to a level that is not adequate to meet the body's needs for tissue oxygenation; the supply does not equal the demand.

Cardiogenic Shock

Cardiogenic shock is caused by a failure of the heart to perform as a pump; it is sometimes referred to as "pump failure."

Neurogenic Shock

Neurogenic shock occurs following sudden vasodilatation in the vascular tree caused by nervous control of the blood vessels. (There is no actual loss of blood volume, but vasomotor tone is diminished).

Vasogenic Shock

In vasogenic shock the vasodilatation that occurs is caused by drugs such as histamine and alcohol, or by histamine released by the body in response to foreign proteins or by toxins from infectious organisms. [6]

ETIOLOGY

Hypovolemic shock may be caused by stressors such as:

Massive gastrointestinal hemorrhage

Blood loss secondary to surgery or trauma

Inadequate fluid intake

Fluid loss accompanying extensive burns, severe vomiting, diarrhea, fistulas, or injudicious use of diuretics

Diabetic shock [4, 5, 6]

Cardiogenic shock may be caused by left ventricular failure secondary to congestive heart failure or acute myocardial infarction, or massive pulmonary embolism. [5, 6]

Neurogenic shock can be caused by stressors such as:

Spinal anesthesia

Brain damage

Drugs that affect the central nervous system (e.g., central nervous system depressants)

Psychic trauma (e.g., worry, fear, emotional tension)[1, 4, 6]

Septic shock (a subclassification of vasogenic shock) is sometimes referred to as bacteremic or endotoxic shock and is a hyperdynamic, hypermetabolic, low vascular resistance state caused by stressors such as: gram-negative infections (e.g., coliform bacilli, meningococci, proteus, salmonella) which are seen in burns, leaking anastomosis with peritonitis, and after endoscopic procedures of the urinary tract. [4]

In anaphylactic shock (another subclassification of vasogenic shock), the client is sensitive to an allergen. The antibody-antigen reaction takes place all through the body immediately after an antigen has entered the circulatory system. [4] Stressors include: drugs, infectious agents, and inhalants.

ASSESSMENT SPECIFIC TO THE ALTERATION

The amount of data collected will depend on the client's condition or response to the shock state. A crisis situation such as shock demands a rapid assessment!

Respiratory System

Assess ventilations to estimate the effectiveness and the amount of respiratory work being done; auscultation is also very important to evaluate breath sounds.

Integumentary System

Assess skin color, temperature, turgor, and moisture. (Diaphoresis may be present because the sweat glands are stimulated by the same nerves that cause vasoconstriction of the blood vessels of the skin.)

Cardiovascular System

Monitor blood pressure, pulse rate and quality, central venous pressure, and pulmonary artery pressure. Blood pressure may be low, normal, or high depending on whether compensatory mechanisms are at work. [7]

Mental Status

Determine the client's level of consciousness and level of anxiety.

Gastrointestinal System

During the abdominal examination, look for signs of distention, tenderness, rigidity, fluid, or masses. The insertion of a nasogastric tube may be necessary to reduce gastric distention and improve venous return.[8]

Musculoskeletal System

Extremities should be examined to detect fractures and/or soft tissue injuries.

Genitourinary System

Monitor and assess urinary output hourly. Output should be approximately 30 to 50 ml/hr.

Laboratory Tests

Initial laboratory values that are essential include:

Hemoglobin

Hematocrit (This may not be a reliable index for measuring blood volume as it is checked before the fluid shift from the interstitial space into the blood stream.)

White blood count

Blood and urinary sugar

Blood urea nitrogen

Arterial blood pH, Pco_2, Po_2, bicarbonate excess or deficit

Serum electrolytes[8]

Chest x-ray and blood cultures also should be obtained.

Classic signs of shock are the signs of increased sympathetic nervous system activity and/or vasoconstriction:

Pallor	Oliguria
Coldness	Collapsed veins
Sweating	Slow capillary filling [8]

The features of septic shock differ somewhat from other
types of shock in that, initially:

The skin is warm, rather than cold.

There is increased body temperature.

Chills, vasodilatation.

Low blood pressure.

Increased metabolic rate.

Leukocytosis.

Skin may be flushed.

Tachycardia and oliguria may also be present. [8]

Biological responses to anaphylactic shock include:

Edema of the face, hands, and other body parts

Wheezing respirations	Rapid, weak pulse
Cyanosis	Falling blood pressure
Dyspnea	Death may follow[8]
Dilated pupils	

CLIENT CARE GOAL

The primary goal in the management of all types of shock
is to increase tissue perfusion by correcting the factors responsible for the hypotension or generalized state of inadequate
circulation.

GENERAL INTERVENTIONS

Position

The client, who is not dyspneic, should be positioned with the head and torso horizontal or slightly elevated with the legs elevated about 20° to 45°, so that cerebral blood flow is not compromised.[6]

Oxygen

Oxygen should be started as soon as possible by mask or nasal catheter/cannula, so that more oxygen is available to the blood. The client's nares should be cleansed and kept free of crusts. Some clients may require the use of mechanical ventilators.

Temperature

The client should be kept comfortably warm, but excess application of heat should be avoided, since heat will cause further vasodilatation.[6]

Analgesics

Severe pain should be controlled promptly. Morphine sulfate may be given intravenously very slowly, but it should not be given to clients who are unconscious, have head injuries, or depressed respirations.

Laboratory Studies

Laboratory tests have been mentioned previously; pulmonary artery wedge pressure is a better indicator of left ventricular function than the central venous pressure.

Parenteral Fluid Therapy

Blood volume should be replaced and maintained. The type of fluid replacement is determined on an individual basis and is based on the type of fluid loss that has occurred.

Vasoactive Drugs

Norepinephrine, metaraminol (Aramine), isoproterenol (Isuprel), and dopamine (Intropin) may be used.

Corticosteroids

The use of corticosteroids in various types of shock syndrome is still controversial. Massive doses of methylprednisolone have been used by some physicians.

Diuretics

Mannitol and furosemide have been recommended in selected clients experiencing oliguria.

SPECIFIC INTERVENTIONS

Hemorrhage and Anemia

Severe anemia must be corrected by replacement with whole blood or packed red cells to prevent hypoxia.

Hypoxia

Oxygen is indicated; the type of therapy is determined by the specific clinical situation and the arterial blood O_2 and CO_2 determinations.

Dehydration

This is corrected by administering the appropriate IV fluids and fluids by mouth as soon as the client is able to take them.

Acid-Base Imbalance

Abnormalities should be corrected promptly, sodium bicarbonate IV may be indicated.

Adrenocortical Failure

Corticosteroids are used specifically to treat the shock of Addison crisis.

Cardiac Disorders

Digitalis may be indicated; atropine may be used to treat bradycardias. The client should be on continuous cardiac monitoring. Intra-aortic balloon counterpulsation has been used in cardiac shock to increase coronary artery perfusion pressure and blood flow and to decrease the left ventricular work load. [2]

Infection

Bacteriologic studies should be initiated before antibiotic therapy is initiated.

Constant monitoring of the client and his responses to therapy is imperative until his condition is stabilized.

COMPLICATIONS

Complications involve progression of shock and death.

REVIEW QUESTIONS

1. Define the state of shock.

2. List four classifications of shock.

3. Describe each of the four classifications of shock.

4. What is the etiology of hypovolemic shock?

5. Name six classic signs of shock.

6. The features of septic shock differ from the other types of shock. What are these differences?

7. List seven possible biological responses to anaphylactic shock.

8. Describe how you would position a client who is in shock.

9. How many blankets should be used to warm a client in shock? Give the rationale for your answer.

10. Urinary output of the client in shock is monitored and assessed hourly. What output in milliliters per hour would be considered acceptable?

REFERENCES

1. Story, J. et al.: Be Alert For Norpace Cardiogenic Shock. Nurses Drug Alert 4 (February 1980): 13.

2. Eckhardt, E.: Intra-Aortic Balloon Counterpulsation in Cardiogenic Shock. Heart Lung 6 (January-February 1977): 93-97.

3. Foster, S. B. and Canty, K.: Pump Failure Following Myocardial Infarction: An Overview. Heart Lung 9 (March-April 1980): 293-297.

4. Guyton, A.: Textbook of Medical Physiology. Philadelphia: W.B. Saunders Co., 1971, pp. 325-336.

5. Jahre, J. et al.: Medical Approach to the Hypotensive Patient and the Patient in Shock. Heart Lung 4 (July-August 1975): 577-587.

6. Luckmann, J. and Sorensen, K.: Medical-Surgical Nursing, A Psychophysiologic Approach. Philadelphia: W.B. Saunders Co., 1974, pp. 264-291, 1980, 230-285.

7. Schumer, W. and Nyhus, L. (Eds.): Treatment of Shock: Principles and Practice. Philadelphia: Lea and Febiger, 1974.

8. Thal, A. et al.: Shock: A Physiological Basis for Treatment. 3rd Ed., Chicago: Year Book Medical Publishers, Inc., 1973.

9. Tharp, G.: Shock: The Overall Mechanisms. Am J Nurs 74 (December 1974): 2208-2211.

CHAPTER 21

THROMBOPHLEBITIS

LEARNING OBJECTIVES

Study of this chapter will enable the reader to:

1. Discuss factors contributing to the development of thrombophlebitis

2. Design nursing interventions to prevent the occurrence of thrombophlebitis

3. Identify clients who are at high risk for the development of thrombophlebitis

4. Describe common symptoms experienced by the client which may indicate the development of thrombophlebitis

5. Appraise the client's physical status regularly to assist in the "early" detection of thrombophlebitis

6. Explain to the client diagnostic tests which are helpful in the diagnosis of thrombophlebitis

7. Formulate a teaching plan to assist the client experiencing an acute episode of thrombophlebitis

8. Propose preventative interventions to high-risk clients and their families

9. Evaluate the effectiveness of medical and nursing interventions on the client's status

10. Revise teaching plans for client education as indicated by client response and physical progress

DESCRIPTION

Thrombophlebitis (phlebitis) is a condition in which there is a partial or complete occlusion of a vein by a thrombus, with secondary inflammation in the wall of the vein.[3] Thrombophlebitis may occur in the deep veins or in the superficial veins. It may arise as a complication of many different clinical conditions.

Basically, three factors contribute to its development:

1. Venous stasis

2. Trauma to the vein

3. Hypercoagulation [7]

The incidence of phlebitis is increased in obese women, the elderly, pregnant women, and women using oral contraceptives. [7]

ETIOLOGY

Many circumstances can contribute to the development of thrombophlebitis such as:

1. Venous stasis which occurs due to immobility following surgery, child birth, prolonged bed rest due to illness, or prolonged sitting with the knees bent sharply

2. Trauma to a vein can be caused by parenteral therapy or may occur during any daily activity [6, 8]

High-risk clients include those who are obese, use estrogen-containing contraceptive pills, have undergone surgery or severe trauma, or have a history of: thrombophlebitis, varicose veins, cardiovascular disease, advanced malignancy, or hypercoagulation. [2, 7]

ASSESSMENT SPECIFIC TO THE ALTERATION

It is estimated that half of the clients with thrombophlebitis have no signs or symptoms in the early stages.[3] Clients who are at high risk should have their lower extremities assessed daily for changes.

SUBJECTIVE DATA

The client's symptoms may include: a dull ache, a tight feeling, or pain in the calf (sometimes in the whole leg) especially when walking. 3

Systemic reaction to the inflammation may cause symptoms such as: headache, malaise, and elevation of temperature. 8

OBJECTIVE DATA

Nursing assessment should include a history, inspection, palpation, and percussion.

History

The client should be questioned about the presence of calf pain, leg pain, redness, swelling, or loss of function in either leg.

Inspection

The feet and legs should be inspected for asymmetric enlargement (especially the calf) and the circumference of both calves should be measured and recorded on a daily basis, using predetermined marked points on the calves for accuracy in measurement. If venous obstruction is severe, the skin may be cyanotic; if reflex arterial spasm is superimposed, the skin may be pale and cool.

Palpation

The affected leg will be warmer to the touch than the unaffected one. The client should be tested for the Homan sign (the foot is forcefully dorsiflexed while the knee is slightly flexed; the test is positive if popliteal and calf pain result); palpation causes discomfort in the affected extremity.

Light Percussion

Tenderness is elicited on light percussion. 3

Diagnostic Tests

New diagnostic tests include:

1. Phlebography is the most accurate and complete method of diagnosis; the extent of the thrombosis is defined by x-ray.

2. Fibrinogen uptake test defines the presence of small thrombi in the calf and allows observation of the thrombotic process for several days; it is the most sensitive test for developing deep venous thrombosis.

3. Ultrasound blood flow detector allows examination of the major veins in an extremity to detect thrombosis; the accuracy of this test is not as great as the others, but it is a useful tool for rapid screening of high-risk clients.

CLIENT CARE GOALS

1. Precautions will be instituted to prevent the occurrence of thrombophlebitis.

2. Early recognition of phlebitis will be accomplished when it does occur.

3. Resolution of thrombi will be promoted by appropriate medical and nursing interventions.

4. Complications will be prevented.

5. Health team members will encourage the client to participate in learning techniques which will prevent the recurrence of thrombophlebitis (i.e., complying with prescribed medical regimen, improving venous return from the lower extremities, precautions to avoid injury to vessels, proper exercises, diet, etc.).

INTERVENTIONS

Prevention

Preventative interventions for clients who are at risk are aimed at:

1. Increasing venous return from the lower extremities

2. Avoiding trauma to vessel walls

3. Correcting hypercoagulation, if present [7]

Active and/or passive leg exercises for approximately 10 minutes every 2 hours will help to increase blood flow and stimulate venous return. When the client is allowed to dangle or sit up in a chair, the nurse should be sure that there is no pressure against the popliteal space from the chair edge or mattress. Any pressure on this space will obstruct venous flow; crossing the legs is not permitted for the same reason.

Clients, who will be sitting up for long periods of time, must be encouraged to exercise leg muscles frequently and to elevate their legs for about 10 minutes each hour. [7] Proper positioning is a must for the client who is on bed rest (i.e., bony prominences should be protected and the entire leg should be supported if elevated, etc.). There continues to be some controversy over the value of using elastic stockings to prevent venous stasis. Properly fitted elastic stockings or elastic bandages are prescribed by some physicans. The Valsalva maneuver increases pressure in the legs and should be avoided. A bulky diet, stool softeners, exercise, and fluid balance can prevent constipation and straining to defecate. [7] Fluid overload or dehydration both contribute to slowing the venous return.

Client education to prevent the development of thrombophlebitis should include:

1. Weight reduction, if the client is obese

2. Termination of smoking cigarettes, since nicotine causes venous constriction

3. Avoidance of constricting garments (i.e., girdles, garters, belts, etc.)

4. Discouraging leg crossing

5. Avoiding vessel injury

6. Obtaining adequate daily exercise [7]

While the client is hospitalized, the nurse should regularly examine his/her legs for signs of thrombophlebitis. The surgical client should have his legs elevated approximately 10° to 20° during long surgical procedures. [3] Postoperative exercises of the legs should start at the close of the operation and be continued for several days. Anticoagulants (low doses of heparin, 5000 units every 12 hours) are occasionally used prophylactically in clients experiencing fractures of the femur, tibia, or in high-risk medical or surgical clients.[3]

Local measures used for the client with acute thrombophlebitis include:

1. Elevation of the legs 15° to 20° with the trunk horizontal

2. After approximately 5 to 10 days (when thrombus is more adherent and the swelling and local symptoms have abated) progressive walking is permitted

3. Elastic stockings or bandages are worn until the swelling tendency has gone.[3]

Medication

Medical interventions for acute thrombophlebitis include the use of heparin initially; later, one of the longer-acting oral anticoagulants such as warfarin or dicumarol can be used.[2,3] A clotting time and prothrombin time are determined before anticoagulation is begun.[3] A clotting time should be done at least every 24 hours ($\frac{1}{2}$ hour before the next scheduled dose of heparin).[3] Protamine sulfate given IV can be used to neutralize heparin if necessary; Phytonadione (Mephyton p.o. or Aquamephyton IV) will counteract the effect of drugs depressing prothrombin. Streptokinase or urokinase (fibrinolytic drugs) are sometimes used to clear occluded leg veins and obstructing pulmonary emboli.[2,3] Anti-inflammatory drugs and analgesics are sometimes used depending on the attending physician's preference.

Surgery

Surgical procedures include: (1) vein ligation when anticoagulant therapy is contraindicated, or in rare cases, (2) femoral vein thrombectomy.[3]

Nursing Management

Nursing management is similar to caring for the client with any peripheral-vascular problem.

Health teaching should include:

1. Preventative measures

2. Compliance with prescribed therapeutic regime

3. Recognizing signs and symptoms of circulatory problems

4. Actions, dosages, methods of administration, side and toxic effects of prescribed drugs

5. The importance of regular medical follow-up

COMPLICATIONS

Pulmonary embolism, recurrent episodes of phlebitis, or chronic venous insufficiency may result. [3]

REVIEW QUESTIONS

1. Define thrombophlebitis.

2. Does thrombophlebitis occur only in the deep veins?

3. What three factors contribute to the development of thrombophlebitis?

4. Which clients are at high risk for developing thrombophlebitis?

5. What symptom does the client with thrombophlebitis frequently complain of?

6. Name the three symptoms which may be caused by a systemic reaction to the inflammation.

7. Explain the following diagnostic tests:

   Phlebography

   Fibrinogen uptake test

   Ultrasound blood flow detector

8. What is Homan sign?

9. What items would you include in your teaching plan when educating the client to prevent the development of thrombophlebitis?

10. Which drug is used to neutralize heparin?

11. List the possible complications of thrombophlebitis.

REFERENCES

1. Bell, R.: A Friend in Need. Nursing Times 75 (May 31, 1979): 912.

2. Douglas, A.: Venous Thrombosis and Pulmonary Embolism: A Disease of Hospitals. Nurs Mirror 147 (October 26, 1978): 44-46.

3. Erskine, J.: Blood Vessels and Lymphatics. In Krupp, M.A. and Chatton, M.J.: Current Medical Diagnosis and Treatment. Los Altos, Calif.: Lange Medical Publications, 1976, pp. 264-269.

4. Fitzmaurice, J.: Venous Thromboembolic Disease: Current Thoughts. Cardiovasc Nurs 14 (January-February 1978): 1-4.

5. Mc Connell, E.: Fitting Antiembolism Stockings. Nursing 78 (September 1978): 67-71.

6. Nyman, J. E.: Thrombophlebitis In Pregnancy. Am J Nurs 80 (January 1980): 90-93.

7. Ryan, R.: Thrombophlebitis: Assessment and Prevention. Am J Nurs 76 (October 1976): 1634-1636.

8. Shafer, K. et al.: Medical-Surgical Nursing. 6th Ed., St. Louis: C.V. Mosby Co., 1975, pp. 392-393.

PART IV

THE PROCESS OF TEACHING AND LEARNING

LEARNING OBJECTIVES

Study of Part IV will enable the reader to:

1. Define terminology in relation to the process of teaching and learning

2. Discuss, in detail, the developmental tasks that must be accomplished during young adulthood, middle-age, and later maturity

3. Detect factors which may negatively affect the adult's learning ability

4. Describe characteristics of adult learners

5. Utilize the steps of the nursing process to resolve problems related to the teaching-learning process

6. Apply the principles of learning in client education

7. Prepare an environment to facilitate the adult client's learning

8. Evaluate teaching effectiveness using established goals

CHAPTER 22

INTRODUCTION TO THE PROCESS OF TEACHING AND LEARNING

It is generally agreed among educators that "education is a lifelong process. " This section of the text focuses on the adult client as a learner. A review of the literature during the past decade reveals the fact that there is a growing body of knowledge and teaching techniques that persons involved in teaching adults can learn to help them become more effective teachers. The literature suggests that there is a distinct and different technology for effective learning to take place in the adult. [9] It behooves members of the nursing profession to keep abreast of the new technologies developed for teaching and learning, so that the teaching role may be performed more effectively. The ultimate goal of teaching the adult client is to assist the client in becoming more competent and responsible for his/her own health care.[10,15] Nurses have the opportunity to facilitate adult learning in both episodic and distributive settings. This section of the text includes a definition of terms, characteristics and developmental tasks of adult learners, the nurse's role as teacher, and the process of teaching and learning (i. e. , principles to consider, conditions facilitating learning, and the nursing process in relation to teaching).

DEFINITION OF TERMS

Behavior: any visible activity manifested by a person (learner). [11]

Concept: a meaningful idea or mental image that is held by a person. [16]

Conceptualization: a complex process that occurs within the learner's mind; it involves six components: (1) perceptions (awareness, insight), (2) emotions (pleasant or unpleasant), (3) verbal symbols (words), (4) integration (process of understanding the similarities, dissimilarities, and operational relationships), (5) generalization (common characteristics of something), and (6) abstraction (a concept is modified and broadened).[16]

Conditioning: a process of learning which can occur on a reflex level (earliest and simplest form of learning) and on a more complex level.[16] The process causes new or modified behavioral responses.

Criterion: a standard by which terminal behavior (learning) is evaluated.[11]

Habits: well-established patterns of behavior developed through practice and repetition.[16]

Imitation: a learning process that may be conscious or unconscious: other people's behavior, mannerisms, attitudes are emulated consciously or unconsciously.[16]

Learning: a process bringing about changes in an individual's response to his environment; learning depends upon the person's physical, mental, and emotional development and upon past and present experiences.[16]

Mental readiness: depends primarily on the individual's state of intellectual development.[16]

Motivation: a force within an individual which influences him to take action; the state of motivation may be aroused by a physical need, an emotion, or an idea.[16]

Objectives: describe the desired outcomes.[11]

Outcomes: final results.

Perception: being aware of the environment; insight, comprehension. (The Merriam-Webster Dictionary, New York: Simon & Schuster, 1974, p. 517.)

Physical readiness: depends on the state of the individual's neuromuscular system; affects the ability to learn physical skills.[16]

Principles: basic laws or truths derived from man's past experience; principles serve to explain known facts in a particular area of knowledge.[16] They are often referred to as "guides to action."

Principles of learning: derived from areas of knowledge related to the ways people act/react in a variety of situations to which they are exposed. [16]

Teaching: the process of helping people to learn; it is the process which facilitates the learning process; it is more than a process of transmitting the culture.

Terminal behavior: the desired behavior the learner should demonstrate at the end of the teaching-learning process. [11]

CHAPTER 23

THE ADULT LEARNER

CHARACTERISTICS OF ADULT LEARNERS

Most practitioners in nursing today subscribe to the belief that each individual is a unique being. It is this "uniqueness" that demands consideration of multiple variables influencing the learning process in the adult learner. Just as a child is not considered to be a "little adult, " the adult should not be treated as merely a "grown up child. " Unlike the child, the adult learner (1) enters the teaching-learning situation voluntarily and (2) brings a multitude of past experiences with him. These experiences will have a positive or a negative influence on whether learning does or does not take place. Adults do not usually continue to pursue learning experiences that are not satisfying to them. The adult acquires knowledge, skills, and values through the various experiences that have taken place in the process of becoming an adult. [3] The adult learner has variable learning needs and will therefore have a diversity of goals as an individual. [3] Another variable to consider when preparing to teach the adult learner is that most adults are generally capable of self-direction if experiences and content are provided.[3] A structured classroom situation usually is not necessary; adults are able to change their behavior (learn) without it.

Dr. Malcolm Knowles, noted author of several books and articles on adult education, has made several assumptions regarding the characteristics of adult learners. He states that as a person develops or attains the desired state of adulthood, he moves from a state of dependence to a state of being self-directed; he gathers a store of experiences which he can use as a resource for future learning, his readiness to learn coincides with the developmental tasks of his social roles, his time perspective changes in that he immediately wishes to apply new knowledge rather than postpone the application of knowledge, and the adult's learning pattern shifts from subject-centeredness to one of centering on a specific problem (problem-solving). [9]

DEVELOPMENTAL TASKS

Young Adult

In general, it can be said that the young adult must achieve the following tasks: he must (1) accept himself and firmly establish his self-concept and body image, (2) establish independence from parents' home and financial assistance, (3) become established in a job or career that offers personal satisfaction, financial independence, and a feeling of societal contribution, (4) learn to value and express love in a responsible manner, (5) establish intimacy with another person (i. e., marriage or friendship), (6) establish and manage a residence, (7) find a social group which is congenial, (8) decide if a family is desired, (9) formulate a philosophy of life, and (10) become involved in community affairs. [14]

Middle-Aged Person

Developmental tasks of the middle-aged person include:

1. Discovering new satisfactions as a marital partner, giving support to the spouse, enjoying mutual activities, and developing a sense of unity and enduring intimacy

2. Helping their children to become happy and responsible adults, showing pride in the children's accomplishments, offering support as needed and accepting their children's friends and marital partner

3. Establishing a pleasant, comfortable home appropriate to personal needs and values; taking pride in self-accomplishments and those of their spouse

4. Finding pleasure and satisfaction in work, growing personally in knowledge and wisdom, balancing work with pleasure and preparing for future retirement

5. Assisting aging parents and parents-in-law, acting as a buffer between the aging parents' demands and the young adults' needs, preparing emotionally for parents' eventual death

6. Attaining social and civic responsibility, keeping informed as a citizen, working cooperatively with others

7. Deriving pleasure and a sense of belonging from actively participating in an organization, assisting in resolving conflict-laden relationships

8. Accepting and adjusting to the physical changes of middle age, maintaining healthful practices and taking pleasure in the bloom of maturity

9. Cherishing old friends and making new ones, enjoying social life with a variety of friends, sharing feelings with at least a few friends

10. Using leisure time creatively and satisfactorily balancing the activities to include active and passive, collective and solitary, service motivated and self-indulgent

11. Continuing to formulate a philosophy of life and religious affiliation, gaining satisfaction from engaging in altruistic activities [14]

Aging Person

Developmental tasks to be achieved by the aging person alone (person in later maturity) or by the aging couple include the need to:

1. Decide how they will spend (live out) the remaining years of life

2. Continue a close relationship with the spouse or significant other

3. Establish a living arrangement (home) which provides a safe and comfortable environment and conforms to their health and financial status

4. Adjust standards of living to limited retirement income

5. Maintain optimum level of health through regular health examinations, dental care, proper diet, exercise, rest, and good personal hygiene

6. Maintain contact with relatives

7. Maintain interest in people other than family members (i.e., community affairs, church, other organizations)

8. Seek out new interests while remaining active in former activities

9. Find meaning in life after retiring from occupation

10. Prepare to face the inevitable death of self and spouse

11. Find comfort in philosophy of life or religion

12. Adjust to the death of spouse.[14]

The nurse educator must assess the degree of success that the adult has experienced in achieving the developmental tasks for his age group. The degree of success or failure in achieving developmental tasks will definitely affect the adult learner's readiness to learn at a given time period.

OTHER SUPPOSITIONS ABOUT ADULT LEARNING

Some individuals hold to the notion that the ability to learn greatly declines as a person grows older. Researchers have shown that the basic ability to learn remains essentially the same throughout the lifespan.[9] Factors affecting learning performance in adults include: (1) lack of confidence in themselves and in their ability to learn, (2) new methods of teaching which are unfamiliar to the adult, (3) physiologic changes which accompany the aging process (i.e., visual and hearing alterations, reactions are slowed, and energy levels are decreased).[9] Another supposition is that learning is an internal process which is controlled by the learner.[9] The adult learner is motivated to learn to the extent that he sees some personal gain or accomplishment through learning a particular skill, procedure, or task.[9] It is generally agreed upon that methods which involve the adult learner most actively in the teaching-learning process produce the greatest learning.

CHAPTER 24

THE NURSE AS TEACHER

ROLES OF THE NURSE TEACHER

The nurse responsible for teaching the adult client functions in several roles as a facilitator, resource person, motivator, climate setter, method selector, provider, implementor, evaluator, and change agent in general. The nurse health educator attempts to satisfy the needs and goals of the adult client, the institution (i. e. , hospital, clinic, health agency), and society (i. e, community, country). As stated previously, this discussion focuses primarily on the adult client. It is beyond the scope of this text to discuss the needs of the institution and society even though these needs are very important and significant considerations.

The nurse may use the steps of the nursing process to resolve any problems related to the teaching-learning process (i. e. , identification of the client's needs, planning, intervention, and evaluation). In the first step of the process, the nurse works directly with the adult client and acts as a facilitator who assists the client to identify his/her own needs in a particular learning situation. This is sometimes referred to as the "assessment phase." Both the nurse and the client first collaborate to determine existing needs and then proceed to establish goals and objectives for the learning experience. The second step of the process is called the "planning phase." Nurse and client agree upon planned experiences that will allow the accomplishment of the goals and objectives to meet identified needs. The nurse accepts responsibility for "setting the climate" or creating conditions that enhance the client's motivation to learn. The role of "method selector" is assumed by the nurse. The nurse's specialized knowledge, experience, and clinical expertise prepare her to select the most appropriate methods to be utilized to obtain the desired outcomes. The "intervention phase" allows the nurse to function in the role of resource person or provider. The nurse provides the client with the resources necessary (human and material) to produce the desired learnings or outcomes. The last phase in the process is the "evaluation phase." The nurse and the client can evaluate the teaching-learning process together to determine if the client's needs were met according to the mutually established goals and objectives (criteria). If the needs were not met, the nurse and client begin the assessment phase again and work through the steps of the problem-solving process until the needs are successfully met. This process also may be used with the client's family or significant others. Research has shown that structured teaching, using specific written guidelines, is more effective than unstructured teaching.[22] The steps of the nursing process and specific teaching guidelines are illustrated in the outline on pages 225 through 258.

Recent literature has popularized the use of the term "change agent" as a role of the nurse. Indeed, the nurse does function as a change agent when she assists the client to change his behavior and to become more competent and responsible for his own health maintenance. This behavior change results in greater satisfaction and productivity for the individual and the society in which he lives.

A SUGGESTED TEACHING OUTLINE FOR THE CLIENT EXPERIENCING A CARDIOVASCULAR ALTERATION

I. Assessment Phase (In preparation for developing a teaching plan)

   A. Identify the client's existing needs in relation to learning

      1. What is the client's concept of the cardiovascular alteration being experienced?

      2. What is the client's reaction to it?

      3. How does the client expect the alteration to alter his lifestyle?

      4. Is the client physically and psychologically ready to learn?

II. Planning Phase

   A. Establish goals and objectives for the learning experience in relation to the data obtained during the assessment phase

   B. Plan teaching experiences, methods, and time periods
to accomplish the goals and objectives (a list of educational materials available from the American Heart
Association is included in the Appendix).

III. Intervention Phase (Specific teaching content)

   A. Discuss the cardiovascular process being experienced

      1. Related anatomy and physiology

   B. Give an overview of the rehabilitation program

   C. Psychosocial aspects

      1. Discuss reactions to the alteration and methods of
adapting (problems related to finances, family,
occupation, community, self-image)

   D. Identify and eliminate or modify risk factors (see
Chapter 1, pp. 4-5)

      1. Prevention of another acute episode

      2. Risk factors that cannot be changed

      3. Risk factors that can be changed

   E. Medications prescribed

      1. What the medication is

      2. Why it is being prescribed

      3. What are the side effects

      4. Drug related interactions as appropriate

      5. Encourage client to seek medical advice if
questions arise

F. Diet

1. Obtain a diet history from the client as a first step in suggesting <u>realistic</u> diet modifications

2. Utilize the dietitian, if available, as a resource person for teaching the client and family

3. Reinforce the dietitian's teaching regarding the reduction of:

Cholesterol and saturated fats	Caffeine
	Sodium intake
Carbohydrates	Excessive alcohol
Calories	consumption

G. Exercise

1. Specific guidelines regarding prescribed progressive activity should be given to client and spouse

H. Special Guidelines

1. Discuss items affecting the client's immediate lifestyle following the acute episode, reviewing:

Warning symptoms (see Chapter 2, pp. 6-10 Warning Signals Cardinal Symptoms/Signs)

Work simplification techniques taught in the hospital

Pacing activities

Specific therapeutic instructions

Follow-up care

I. Sexual Activities

1. This topic may not be brought up spontaneously by the client, but it should be understood (see Chapter 6, pp. 58-61 for specific guidelines for the cardiac client)

J. Follow-Up Care Posthospitalization

　　1. Definite plan is needed

　　2. Encourage client to seek medical advice for any questions/concerns arising during the interim

　　3. Follow-up visits offer an excellent opportunity for answering questions and reinforcing teaching

IV. Evaluation Phase

A. Develop an evaluation tool

B. Nurse and client evaluate the teaching-learning process together to determine if the client's needs were met according to the mutually established goals and objectives

C. If "needs" were not met, the nurse and the client begin the assessment phase again and work through the steps of the problem-solving process again [16, 22]

CHAPTER 25

THE PROCESS OF TEACHING AND LEARNING

PRINCIPLES OF LEARNING (GUIDES TO ACTION)

Principles of learning include the following:

1. The adult client (learner) must be able to receive messages from the world around him: "Perception" is necessary if the client is to learn.[16] Three steps are involved in perception: (a) sense organs must receive a stimulus, (b) the stimulus (impulse) must be transferred to a sensory area in the brain by the afferent nervous system, and (c) the brain must interpret the stimulus as a sensation of sight, sound, taste, odor, or touch.[16] Errors in perception frequently occur if the sensory system is not functioning properly or if the client is experiencing an intense emotion such as fear.[16]

2. Conditioning has an effect on learning. Conditioning may have a positive or negative effect on learning. The nurse educator who understands the process of conditioning will plan experiences so that the positive responses which will benefit the client are reinforced; undesirable responses will be eliminated.[16]

3. Trial and error are ways of learning; however, time and energy are often wasted in this method. The nurse can use her expertise to suggest appropriate ways for the client to master skills; the nurse's encouragement and approval also help to reinforce learning.[16]

4. Imitation plays a role in learning. The process of imitation may be conscious or unconscious. Demonstration is often an effective method of teaching—the learner imitates the teacher's behavior until he/she is able to perform the task adequately.[16]

259

5. The learning process involves the development of concepts (see Chapter 22 for the definition of concepts and conceptualization).[16] The nurse must assume responsibility to determine if the client's concepts regarding specific areas are valid.

6. Individuals must be motivated if learning is to take place.[16] The process of motivation takes place within the individual. The client must want to learn; the client cannot be forced to learn something that he/she does not want to learn. As mentioned previously, the adult is a voluntary learner. If he/she does not wish to learn, he/she will remove him/herself from the learning situation physically or mentally. Physical and emotional stresses must be removed if the client's motivation is to be directed toward learning.[16] The desire to learn must be stronger than other drives.[16] If the adult client shows no interest in learning, the nurse has a responsibility to try to discover the reason for the indifference and plan to correct the situation.[16] Why are some individuals motivated to learn while others are not? Some people are naturally curious and wish to learn as much as possible regarding their condition (alteration); some are impressed with the importance of maintaining health, and those who are ill or have been ill in the past, wish to regain their health and maintain it. The nurse must initially establish rapport with the client and establish a trusting relationship before he/she can begin the "assessment phase" of identification of learning needs and planning the learning experience.

7. The client must be physically and mentally ready to learn (often referred to as "readiness to learn" or "readiness for learning"). The client may not be developmentally ready to learn; normal growth, development, and maturation are prerequisites for learning. In every situation, content must be adapted or geared to the client's level of development.[16] Alterations of the neuromuscular system can affect the learning of skills and procedures temporarily or permanently.[16] In the case of permanent alterations or deficits, the nurse must teach the client's family/significant others rather than the client.

8. Active participation is the key to effective learning. The more the adult client participates, the more he is likely to learn.[16]

9. New learning is influenced by previous knowledge and

experience. 16 To be mastered, skills should progress from simple to complex. 16 The nurse teacher should limit teaching to the essentials that the client must know. Exotic details lead to confusion on the part of the client and his family.

10. Emotions affect learning. An extreme emotional climate results in little effective learning. 16 A small or moderate amount of anxiety may motivate the individual or enhance learning; extremes are detrimental to learning (i.e., the client experiencing fear, anger, pain is usually very unreceptive to new learning; the emotions or sensations must be relieved first).

11. Repetition facilitates learning. Habit formation facilitates learning. 16

12. Learning is reinforced when satisfaction is present. If we enjoy what we are doing, we are more likely to continue doing it. 16 The rewards may be internal (within the client) or external (from others). Moderate amounts of dissatisfaction may be a learning stimulus. 16

OPTIMAL CONDITIONS FOR LEARNING

Before initiating the steps of the teaching-learning process, the nurse teacher attends to preparing the environment to facilitate the adult client's learning. The adult client should be experiencing physical comfort (comfortable seating arrangements, ventilation, temperature, lighting, etc.), mutual trust, respect, and a feeling that his/her ideas can be freely expressed. 9 Other optimal conditions for learning include: (1) the adult learner has defined his own needs and has specific goals to be accomplished, (2) the adult learner accepts responsibility for his/her own learning, (3) the adult learner actively participates in learning, (4) the experience of the adult learner is utilized in the teaching-learning process, (5) the adult learner experiences a sense of satisfaction as goal accomplishment is approached. 9

Educating the adult client is not a luxury; it is a necessity if clients are to receive the greatest possible benefit from today's knowledge of treatment, prevention, and control of disease. 22 The client has a right to information that will enhance his efforts to return to his former lifestyle; the professional nurse has an obligation to provide it.

REVIEW QUESTIONS TO PART IV

1. Define the following terms:

Behavior	Motivation
Concept	Objectives
Conceptualization	Outcomes
Conditioning	Perception
Criterion	Physical readiness
Habits	Principles
Imitation	Principles of learning
Learning	Teaching
Mental readiness	Terminal behavior

2. Describe the developmental tasks that must be accomplished by the young adult, the middle-aged person, and the aging person.

3. Does the <u>ability</u> to learn decline as a person grows older?

4. Name <u>three</u> factors which may affect the learning performance in adults.

5. What are the steps of the nursing process that can be applied to the teaching-learning process?

6. The nurse functions in many roles. Name <u>nine</u> of them.

7. Describe the assessment phase, planning phase, intervention phase and evaluation phase of the teaching-learning process.

8. Name the three steps involved in "perception. "

9. What role does "imitation" play in the learning process?

10. Can the adult be forced to learn?

11. What role does <u>active participation</u> play in learning?

12. Name <u>five</u> optimal conditions for learning.

REFERENCES TO PART IV

1. Bennis, W. , Benne, K. , Chin, R. : The Planning of Change.
   New York: Holt, Rinehart and Winston, 1968.

2. Bloom, B. : Taxonomy of Educational Objectives. New
   York: David McKay Co. , Inc. , 1966 (reprint).

3. Del Bueno, D. J. : Competency Based Education. Nurse
   Educator 3 (May-June 1978): 10-14.

4. Gronlund, N. E. : Stating Behavioral Objectives for Classroom Instruction. New York: Macmillan Co. , 1970.

5. Havighurst, R. J. and Orr, B. : Adult Education and Adult
   Needs. Boston: Center for the Study of Liberal Education
   for Adults, 1956.

6. Highet, G. : The Art of Teaching. New York: Alfred A.
   Knopf, Inc. , 1963.

7. Hilgard, E. J. : Theories of Learning and Instruction.
   Chicago: University of Chicago Press, 1964.

8. Jones, P. and Oertel, W. : Developing Patient Teaching
   Objectives and Techniques: A Self-Instructional Program.
   Nurse Educator II (September-October 1977): 3-17.

9. Knowles, M. S. : The Modern Practice of Adult Education.
   4th printing. New York: Association Press, 1973.

10. Linde, B. and Janz, N. : Effect of a Teaching Program on
    Knowledge and Compliance of Cardiac Patients. Nurs Res
    28 (September-October 1979): 282-286.

11. Mager, R. F. : Preparing Instructional Objectives. Bel-
    mont, Calif: Fearon Publishers, Inc. , 1962.

12. Maslow, A. H. : Motivation and Personality. New York:
    Harper and Brothers, 1954.

13. Mico, P. and Ross, H.: Health Education and Behavioral Science. Oakland, Calif.: Third Associates, Inc., 1975, pp. 55-57.

14. Murray, R. and Zentner, J.: Nursing Assessment and Health Promotion through the Lifespan. Englewood Cliffs, N.J.: Prentice-Hall, Inc., 1975.

15. Braithwaite, J.D. and Morton, B.: Patient Education for Blood Pressure Control. Nurs C N Am 16 (June 1981): 321-329.

16. Pohl, M.: The Teaching Function of the Nurse Practitioner. Dubuque, Iowa: William C. Brown Co. Publishers, 1973.

17. Raymer, M.: Improving Patient Teaching With An All-In-One Program. Nursing 80 (August 1980): 18-19.

18. Redman, B.K.: The Process of Patient Teaching in Nursing. St. Louis: C.V. Mosby Co., 1972.

19. Schrank, J.: Teaching Human Beings. Boston: Beacon Press, 1972.

20. Skinner, B.F.: The Technology of Teaching. New York: Appleton-Century-Crofts, 1968.

21. Weisgerber, R.A.: Perspectives in Individualized Learning. Itasca, Ill.: F.E. Peacock Publishers, Inc., 1971.

22. Winslow, E.H. (Ed.): Teaching and Rehabilitating the Cardiac Patient. Nurs C N Am 11 (June 1976): 219-220, 242-249.

APPENDIX

It is intended that the drug tables included in this section be
used as a quick reference guide for the reader and not as a
reference for the prescription of drugs.

ANTIANGINAL AGENTS

Agent/Trade Name	Usual Adult Dose	Mechanism of Action	Side Effects
Nitroglycerin (Nitroglycerin, Nitrostat)	Sublingual (SL): 0.3-0.6 mg p.r.n. (0.3 mg = 1/200 gr 0.4 mg = 1/150 gr 0.6 mg = 1/100 gr)	Causes relaxation of smooth muscle of the vascular system, which in turn lowers the arterial systolic pressure. Because left ventricle pumps against a lower systolic pressure, myocardial oxygen consumption is decreased Remarks: 1. Nitroglycerin supply should be renewed every 3 months to ensure potency 2. Tablets should be stored in their original brown container with lid tightly closed 3. Cotton should not be placed in the container because it absorbs nitroglycerin	Flushing, headache, dizziness, postural hypotension, local burning sensation in the oral cavity
Nitroglycerin Ointment 2%	Dosage is determined individually for each client and is based on baseline heart rate and blood pressure values	It has a longer action time than Nitroglycerin SL	Same
Nitroglycerin (sustained release) (Nitro-Bid, Nitrospan)	P.O.: 1.3-6.5 mg 1 capsule every 8-12 hr, except Nitrospan: 1 capsule every 12 hr	Sustained release action	Same

ANTIANGINAL AGENTS (Cont.)

Agent/Trade Name	Usual Adult Dose	Mechanism of Action	Side Effects
Isosorbide dinitrate (Isordil, Sorbitrate)	SL or slowly chewed: 2.5-5 mg p.r.n. or every 2-3 hr, P.O.: 5-30 mg 4 times/day	Action similar to nitroglycerin, but onset of action is slower (3 to 5 minutes)	Same
Propranolol (Inderal)	P.O.: 10-80 mg every 6 hr	Blocks sympathetic nerve stimulation (decreases heart rate), atrioventricular conduction and myocardial tension resulting in decreased myocardial O_2 consumption Remarks: 1. Dosage should be reduced gradually before discontinuing the drug 2. Drug is contraindicated if the client has: bronchial asthma, allergic rhinitis, sinus bradycardia, heart block, cardiogenic shock, right ventricular failure secondary to pulmonary hypertension or congestive heart failure 3. Use with caution in diabetes: can cause hypoglycemia and its side effects 4. If the systolic blood pressure is below 90 mm Hg, consult with the physician before administering	Nausea, vomiting, diarrhea, or constipation, lightheadedness, rash, depression, weakness, fatigue, drug fever, sore throat, visual disturbances, hallucinations, insomnia, short-term memory loss, disorientation to time and place, transient alopecia (see p.275 for additional untoward effects)

ANTIARRHYTHMIC DRUGS

Indications	Dosage	Therapeutic Blood Level	Major Effects	Untoward Effects	Treatment of Toxicity
Digitalis (Half-Life 34 hr)					
Atrial flutter, atrial fibrillation, paroxysmal atrial tachycardia (PAT)	P.O. and IV for digitalization: 0.75-1.5 mg over 24 hr for maintenance: 0.125-0.5 mg/day	0.5-2.0 μg/ml	Increase in contractility, decrease in heart rate, decrease in atrial automaticity, increase in AV node refractoriness, increase in ventricular automaticity ECG: Increase in PR interval, QRS unchanged, decrease in T wave amplitude, ST segment shortened and depressed	Headache, dizziness, nausea/vomiting, diarrhea, fatigue, weakness, visual disturbances Arrhythmias: PAT with heart block, ventricular ectopy, junctional rhythms, AV block, ventricular tachycardia or fibrillation, sinus arrest	Discontinue drug, correct hypokalemia, correct hypoxia Drugs: Phenytoin, Lidocaine, Propranolol Recent approaches: cholestyramine (binds digoxin in GI tract), digoxin-specific antibodies
Lidocaine (xylocaine) (Half-Life 15-30 min)					
Ventricular ectopy, ventricular tachycardia	IV bolus: 50-100 mg followed by a constant infusion of 2-4 mg/min	1.2-6.0 μg/ml	Decrease in ventricular automaticity and excitability (local "anesthetic" effect) stabilizing of cell membranes, decrease in conductivity,	Dizziness, confusion, drowsiness, tinnitus, nausea, irritability, respiratory depression, focal seizures, hypotension, convulsions, bradycardia, sinoatrial arrest, heart block	Discontinue drug diazepam (Valium) to control convulsions

ANTIARRHYTHMIC DRUGS (Cont.)

Indications	Dosage	Therapeutic Blood Level	Major Effects	Untoward Effects	Treatment of Toxicity
			increase in ventricular fibrillation threshold ECG: No change in PR, QRS, or QT interval		

Procainamide (Pronestyl) (Half-Life 3 hr)

| Ventricular ectopy, ventricular tachycardia, supraventricular tachycardia | IV: 50-100 mg every 5 min up to a maximum dose of 1 gm followed by a 2-6 mg/min drip
IM: 0.5-1 gm every 4-6 hr
P.O.: 1 gm initially, then 250-500 mg every 3-4 hr | 3-10 µg/ml | Increase in atrial refractoriness, decrease in automaticity, decrease in excitability, decrease in conductivity, decrease in contractility

ECG:
Increase in PR interval, increase in QRS width, increase in QT interval | Thrombocytopenia, worsening heart failure, nausea/vomiting, anorexia, depression, weakness, agranulocytosis, anaphylaxis

Systemic lupus-like syndrome, arthralgia, fever, skin rash, hepatomegaly, increase in ANA titer

Arrhythmias:
Heart block, electrical asystole, ventricular fibrillation | Discontinue drug, vasopressors for decrease in BP, direct counter shock for unstable rhythms |

Quinidine Sulfate (Half-Life 4-6 hr)

Atrial flutter, atrial fibrillation, paroxysmal atrial tachycardia, ventricular ectopy, ventricular tachycardia	P.O.: 200-400 mg every 4-6 hr	2.6 µg/ml	Decrease in automaticity, decrease in excitability, decrease in conductivity, decrease in contractility, increase in AV node conduction ECG: Increase in PR interval or no change, increase in QRS width, increase in QT interval	Hypersensitivity, GI distress, anorexia, thrombocytopenia, hypotension, Cinchonism: Tinnitus, blurred vision, Arrhythmias: Sinus arrest, SA block, AV block, ventricular tachycardia, ventricular fibrillation, asystole	Discontinue drug, vasopressors for decrease in BP, direct counter shock for unstable rhythms

Phenytoin (Dilantin) (Half-Life 24 hr)

Arrhythmias associated with digitalis toxicity: paroxysmal atrial tachycardia, ventricular ectopy, ventricular tachycardia	IV: 50-100 mg every 5 min up to 1 gm total dose P.O.: 1 gm loading dose every 24 hr then 300-500 mg/day	10-18 µg/ml	Decrease in automaticity, decrease in excitability, increase in AV conduction ECG: Decrease in PR interval or no change, decrease in QT interval or no change	Hypersensitivity, drowsiness, ataxia, nausea, blurred vision, nystagmus, blood dyscrasias, gum hyperplasia, hypotension Arrhythmias: Ventricular fibrillation, ventricular standstill	Discontinue drug

ANTIARRHYTHMIC DRUGS (Cont.)

Indications	Dosage	Therapeutic Blood Level	Major Effects	Untoward Effects	Treatment of Toxicity
Bretylium (Bretylol) (Half-Life 8-10 hr)					
Refractory ventricular tachycardia/ fibrillation	IV: Initial dose: 5-10 mg/kg body wt, repeat in 1-2 hr IV or IM maintenance: 5 mg/ kg every 6-8 hr or a 1-2 mg/min drip	Not established	Increase in contractility, increase in automaticity, increase in ventricular fibrillation threshold ECG: No change	Hypotension, nausea/vomiting, increase in sensitivity to catecholamines	Discontinue drug, IV fluids and vasopressors for decrease in BP
Disopyramide (Norpace) (Half-Life 6 hr)					
Ventricular ectopy, ventricular tachycardia	P.O.: 200-300 mg loading dose followed by 100-200 mg every 6 hr	2-6 μg/ml	Decrease in contractility, decrease in automaticity, decrease in conductivity, increase in AV node conduction, decrease in excitability ECG: Increase in PR interval or no change, increase in QRS width, increase in QT interval	Dry mouth, aggravation of glaucoma, urinary retention, blurred vision, GI distress, headache, fatigue, hypotension, heart block, "Norpace-syncope"	Discontinue drug

Propranolol (Inderal) (Half-Life IV 2-3 hr, P.O. 3-6 hr)

| Sinus tachycardia, atrial flutter, atrial fibrillation, paroxysmal atrial tachycardia, digitalis-induced ventricular arrhythmias, ventricular ectopy, ventricular tachycardia, ventricular fibrillation | IV: 1 mg/min up to a total of 5-7 mg P.O.: 10-200 mg 3-4 times/day | Not established; 50-100 mg/ml required for beta-adrenergic blockade | Decrease in heart rate, decrease in contractility, decrease in automaticity, decrease in excitability, decrease in conductivity, increase in AV node refractoriness, decrease in blood pressure

ECG: Increase in PR interval or no change, QRS no change, decrease in QT interval or no change | Bradycardia, hypotension, congestive heart failure, bronchospasm, fatigue, dizziness, cold feet, insomnia, GI distress, heart block, hyperglycemia, hypoglycemia, depression | Discontinue drug, atropine (isoproterenol) Isuprel for bradycardia, vasopressors for decrease in BP, aminophylline for bronchospasm, digitalis/diuretics for heart failure |

ANTICOAGULANTS

Agent/Trade Name	Usual Adult Dose	Mechanism of Action	Side Effects
Heparin sodium (Lipo Hepin, Panheparin)	Subcutaneous: Initially: 10,000-20,000 units, then: 8,000-10,000 units every 8 hr or 12,000-20,000 units every 12 hr Intermittent IV: Initially 10,000 units, then 5,000-10,000 units every 4-6 hr Continuous IV: Initial loading dose of 5,000 units direct IV before continuous infusion, 20,000-40,000 units in D5W or isotonic saline to infuse in a 24-hr period	Prevents clot extension directly by retarding the formation of fibrin (therefore, blood clotting time is prolonged) Remark: Heparin sodium toxicity is treated with the heparin antagonist protamine sulfate	GI bleeding, wound hematoma, hemarthrosis, adrenal hemorrhage, hypersensitivity reaction: chills, fever, urticaria, osteoporosis and suppression of renal function after prolonged therapy; transient alopecia, aldosterone suppression
Acetylsalicylic acid (Aspirin, A.S.A.)	600 mg b.i.d.	Antiplatelet agent: prevents the primary process of platelet aggregation Remark: Aspirin potentiates the action of coumarin and should be avoided when coumarin is being used	Rapid, deep breathing, nausea, vomiting, vertigo, tinnitus, flushing, increased perspiration

| Warfarin (Coumadin sodium, Panwarfin) | Initially 10-50 mg divided over a period of 2-4 days (avg. dose 10 mg) Maintenance dose range: 2-10 mg depending on pro-thrombin time determina-tions | Interferes with the synthesis of clotting factors; acts in the liver to inhibit vitamin K in the production of prothrombin and several other clotting fac-tors

Remarks:
Some commonly used drugs potentiate the action of cou-marin in man and should be avoided when coumarin is used:
quinidine
chloral hydrate
phenylbutazone
salicylates
indomethacin
phenytoin
tolbutamide
[The antidote for Warfarin Sodium toxicity is vitamin K1 (phytonadione)] | Hemorrhage, GI bleeding, he-maturia, nephropathy, blood dyscrasias, rash, pruritis, urticaria, alopecia, fever, sore throat, petechiae, ecchymosis, bleeding from mucus mem-branes, wound hemorrhage, paralytic ileus, uterine bleed-ing, epistaxis, cerebral hem-orrhage, fetal hemorrhage (if given during pregnancy)

Prothrombinopenic state in an infant if given to a lactating mother |

DRUGS COMMONLY USED IN HYPERTENSION

Agent/Trade Name	Usual Adult Dose	Mechanism of Action	Side Effects
Thiazides			
Chlorothiazide (Diuril)	500-1,000/day p.o. or IV 50-100 mg/day p.o.	1. Prevent Na^+ and H_2O reabsorption in the distal tubules 2. Promote K^+ excretion 3. Potentiate other antihypertensive drugs	1. Hypokalemia 2. Hyperuricemia 3. Hyperglycemia 4. Hyponatremia (rare) 5. Skin rashes 6. Hepatic coma (cirrhosis)
Hydrochlorothiazide (Exidrix HydroDIURIL, Oretic)			
Chlorthalidone (Hygroton)	25-100 mg/day p.o.		
Loop Diuretics			
Furosemide (Lasix)	40-80 mg/day p.o.	1. Depresses NaCl reabsorption in the ascending loop of Henle 2. Promotes K^+ excretion 3. Action rapid, but of short duration	Loop diuretics have essentially the same side effects as the thiazides, but the effects are more intensified
Potassium-Sparing Diuretics			
Spironolactone (Aldactone)	50-100 mg/day p.o.	1. Is an aldosterone antagonist, therefore prevents reabsorption of Na^+ and H_2O, and hinders the excretion of K^+ by the kidney 2. Potentiates action of other diuretics	1. Nausea 2. Gynecomastia-males 3. Menometrorrhagia in women Remarks: 1. Has been shown to be a tumorigen in chronic toxicity

Drug	Dosage	Action	Side Effects
Triamterene (Dyrenium)	100-300 mg/day p.o.	1. Acts on the distal tubule to inhibit reabsorption of Na^+ ions in exchange for potassium and hydrogen	studies in rats - unnecessary use of this drug should be avoided 2. Should be given with meals to prevent nausea 1. Hyperkalemia may occur if renal function is impaired or if there is a sudden intake of K^+ rich foods

Beta Blockers

Drug	Dosage	Action	Side Effects
Propranolol (Inderal)	40-480 mg/day	1. Nonselective beta-blockers which can occupy beta receptor sites in cardiac, arterial, and bronchial tissue preventing stimulation of the organs 2. Inhibit renin secretion	1. May aggravate or precipitate CHF in certain clients with decreased cardiac reserve 2. Other possible effects: diarrhea, constipation, mental depression, insomnia, nightmares, severe bradycardia 3. May mask signs of hypoglycemia 4. May cause bronchospasm in some people 5. May aggravate Raynaud phenomenon or intermittent claudication
Nadolol (Corgard)	40-160 mg/day		1. Eosinophilia

DRUGS COMMONLY USED IN HYPERTENSION (Cont.)

Agent/Trade Name	Usual Adult Dose	Mechanism of Action	Side Effects
Metoprolol tartrate (Lopressor)	100-200 mg/day	1. Cardioselective beta-blocker that blocks beta receptors in the heart, decreasing cardiac contractility and CO 2. Has less effect upon bronchial smooth muscle, and peripheral vascular tone than a nonselective beta-blocker	1. Effects about the same as above except that it is less apt to precipitate or aggravate Raynaud phenomenon or intermittent claudication in patients with peripheral vascular disease
Adrenergic Blockers			
Reserpine (Serpasil)	0.1-0.25 mg/day p.o.	1. Decrease norepinephrine concentration centrally and at postganglionic sites 2. Minor effects on BP when used alone, but is more effective when used in combination with diuretics	1. Increased appetite 2. Nasal congestion 3. Diarrhea 4. Gastric hyperacidity 5. Lethargy, drowsiness 6. Mental depression Remarks: 1. Contraindicated in clients having a history of depression 2. Recent concern regarding carcinogenic effects in animals. This cause and effect relationship has not been demonstrated in humans as yet

Clonidine
(Catapres)

0.1-1.0 mg/day

1. Stimulates alpha receptors in the brain thereby inhibiting the sympathetic vasomotor center and sympathetic outflow

1. Drowsiness
2. Dry mouth
3. Fatigue
4. Constipation
5. Dizziness
6. Inhibition of ejaculation

Remarks:
1. If medication is stopped abruptly, rebound hypertension can occur

Methyldopa
(Aldomet)

500-2,000 mg/day p.o.

1. Interferes with the synthesis of norepinephrine by substituting methyldopa for dopa: methyl-norepinephrine is formed
2. This replaces norepinephrine centrally and in the neuroeffector fibers is often referred to as a "false transmitter"
3. Results in a lowered BP
4. Renin release is blocked

1. Bradycardia
2. Decreased cardiac output
3. Drowsiness
4. Fatigue
5. Postural hypotension
6. Nasal congestion
7. Impotence
8. Diarrhea
9. Dry mouth
10. Mental depression

Remarks:
1. Contraindicated in liver disease
2. May cause positive Coombs test; hemolytic anemia is rare

DRUGS COMMONLY USED IN HYPERTENSION (Cont.)

Agent/Trade Name	Usual Adult Dose	Mechanism of Action	Side Effects
Guanethidine sulfate (Ismelin)	10-100 mg/day	1. A potent sympatholytic agent with a long duration of action 2. Blocks transmission of impulses along the neuron resulting in depletion of stores of norepinephrine in granules of the postganglionic nerve fibers by blocking the reuptake and release of norepinephrine	1. Orthostatic hypotension 2. Decreased cardiac output may lead to increase in plasma volume and CHF 3. Diarrhea 4. Ejaculatory impotence
Agents Acting Directly on Vascular Smooth Muscle (Vasodilators)			
Hydralazine hydrochloride (Apresoline)	50-300 mg/day p.o.	1. Causes arteriolar dilatation 2. Causes reflex cardiac stimulation 3. Renal vascular resistance is reduced (an advantage for the client in renal failure) 4. Used with an oral diuretic and a sympathetic blocking agent	1. Headache 2. Tachycardia 3. Palpitations 4. Fever 5. Nausea 6. Vomiting 7. Flushing 8. May aggravate CHF or angina 9. Lupus-like reaction and arthritis occur rarely

Minoxidil (Loniten)	10-40 mg/day	1. Very potent vasodilator with above actions; however should only be used if the client is resistant to other drugs	1. Tachycardia 2. Palpitations 3. Edema 4. Hirsutism 5. Breast tenderness 6. Pericardial effusion possible
Other New <u>Antihypertensives</u>			
Prazosin (Minipress)	10-15 mg/day (Usually start with 2 mg/day x 3 days and gradually increase)	1. Blocks peripheral sympathetic nerve activity by interfering with postsynaptic alpha receptors: results in peripheral vascular dilatation	1. Syncope may occur with initial dose 2. Postural dizziness 3. Palpitations 4. Headache 5. Drowsiness 6. Weakness 7. Nausea 8. GI symptoms

DRUGS COMMONLY USED IN HYPERTENSIVE EMERGENCIES

Agent/Trade Name	Usual Adult Dose	Mechanism of Action	Side Effects
Drugs That Act on Vascular Smooth Muscle Directly			
Diazoxide (Hyperstat)	300 mg IV rapidly (15 sec) to avoid protein binding and non-availability of the drug at receptor sites	1. Directly dilates peripheral resistance vessels 2. Increase cardiac output and heart rate while maintaining renal blood flow 3. It has little effect on capacitance vessels; does not interfere with sympathetic reflexes	Hyperglycemia, flushing, nausea, vomiting
Sodium nitroprusside (Nipride)	25-300 μg/min IV drip	1. Dilate both resistance and capacitance vessels 2. BP is lowered by decreasing both the peripheral vascular resistance and the CO; heart rate increases slightly Remark: Due to the light sensitivity of sodium nitroprusside, the IV solution and the tubing should be wrapped in foil; the solution should be discarded in 4 hr if unused	Nausea, vomiting, muscle twitching, possible thiocynanate toxicity, can cause a precipitous fall in blood pressure if infused too rapidly

Hydralazine (Apresoline)	10-20 mg IM or IV	1. Directly dilates peripheral resistance vessels	Palpitations, tachycardia, flushing, angina, headache, occasionally aggravates/precipitates coronary insufficiency and CHF when administered alone

Drugs That Act on the Sympathetic Nervous System

Trimethaphan (Arfonad)	0.5-1.0 mg/min initially; it is increased gradually until the BP falls 20 mm Hg or more	1. Acts primarily by blocking neural transmission in autonomic ganglia 2. Dilates both capacitance and resistance vessels and decreases cardiac output	Urinary retention, orthostatic hypotension, dry mouth, loss of accommodation, ileus
Phentolamine (Regitine)	5 mg IM or IV (increased dosages may be needed)	1. Competes with norepinephrine for alpha-adrenergic receptors; it is a competitive inhibitor of norepinephrine	Flushing, tachycardia, cardiac arrhythmias possible, nausea, vomiting, diarrhea, weakness, dizziness, orthostatic hypotension, nasal stuffiness
Methyldopa (Aldomet)	250-1,000 mg IV	1. Reduces peripheral vascular resistance with only a modest fall in cardiac output; no reduction in blood flow	Drowsiness, dryness of mouth, liver abnormalities

DRUGS COMMONLY USED IN HYPERTENSIVE EMERGENCIES (Cont.)

Agent/Trade Name	Usual Adult Dose	Mechanism of Action	Side Effects
Reserpine (Serpasil)	1-5 mg IM or IV	1. Depletes stores of catecholamines generally and of serotonin especially from platelets and the CNS	Drowsiness, stupor, coma, bradycardia with high doses, may activate a latent peptic ulcer
Diuretics			
Furosemide (Lasix) Ethacrynic acid (Edecrin)	40-80 mg IM or IV 50-100 mg IV slowly	Both potent diuretics which block NaCl reabsorption in the ascending loop of Henle	Severe dehydration after repeated high doses, cramps, hypokalemia

A LIST OF MATERIALS FOR THE PUBLIC*
Produced by the
American Heart Association

About Your Heart and Your Bloodstream

After a Heart Attack

Alta Presion Arterial
(High Blood Pressure)

American Heart Association AD HOC Committee on
Cigarette Smoking and Cardiovascular Disease

American Heart Association Cookbook, 2nd Edition

American Heart Association Has Something
Important to Say

Anti-Smoking Poster—General Audience

Anti-Smoking Poster—Pre-Natal Audience

Anti-Smoking Poster—Teenage Audience

Anti-Smoking Poster—Young Parents Audience

Asociacion Americana del Corazon Tiene Algo
Importante que Decir
(American Heart Association Has Something
Important to Say)

Body Language—How Your Body Warns You of an
Impending Stroke and What to do About It

Case for Biomedical Research

Case of the Sudden Sickness—A Mystery for
Doctor Truso

Cinco Datos Que Usted Necesita Saber Acerca
de Las Enfermedades del Corazon
(Five Facts You Should Know About Heart Disease)

Circulatory System—Chart

Circulatory System—Diagram

Coma Bien, Pero con Sabiduria
(Eat Well, But Eat Wisely)

*Reproduced with permission from the American Heart Association.

A LIST OF MATERIALS FOR THE PUBLIC (Cont.)

Cooking Without Your Salt Shaker

Datos Sobre Derrames Cerebrales (Facts About Strokes)

Diez Mandamientos para El Paciente con Alta Presion Arterial-Tarjeta (10 Commandments for the Patient with High Blood Pressure)

E Is for Exercise

Eat Well but Eat Wisely to Reduce Your Risk of Heart Attack

Emergency Action-Wallet Card

En Caso de Emergencia-Tarjeta (In Case of Emergency-Wallet Card)

Fact Sheet on Heart Attack, Stroke, and Risk Factors

Facts About Congestive Heart Failure

Facts About Strokes

Feeling Great? Have Your Blood Pressure Checked-Poster

First Aid for Choking-Wallet Card

Five Facts You Should Know About Heart Disease

Guide for Teachers-Children with Heart Disease

Guide for Weight Reduction

Healthy Eating for Teenagers-An Eye to the Future

Heart and Blood Vessels

Heart Attack

Heart Attack-How to Reduce Your Risk

Heart Puzzle

Heart Quiz

High Blood Pressure

High Blood Pressure?-Poster

High Blood Pressure and How to Control It

How Can High Blood Pressure Hurt You?

How the Doctor Examines Your Heart

How to Stop Smoking

If Your Blood Pressure Is Up Don't Let It Get You Down-Poster

If Your Child Has A Congenital Heart Defect

Innocent Heart Murmurs in Children

Inside the Cardiac Care Unit—A Guide for the Patient and Family

Living with Angina

Living with Your Pacemaker

May Is High Blood Pressure Month—Poster

Medicine Cabinet Sticker

No Se Arriesgue A un Ataque Cardiaco (Why Risk Heart Attack)

Nutrition Labeling Food Selection Hints for Fat-Controlled Meals

Older Person's Guide to Cardiovascular Health

Portable Quizamatic Exhibit

Protect Your Child's Heart

Proteja El Corazon de Sus Hijos (Protect Your Child's Heart)

Quizamatic Cards

Recipes for Fat-Controlled, Low-Cholesterol Meals

Reduce Your Risk of Heart Attack

Safe Work Load for Farmers with Heart Disease

Safeguarding Your Heart During Pregnancy

Save Food $ and Help Your Heart

Seven Hopeful Facts About Stroke

Siete Hechos Sobre Ataques o Derrames Cerebrales (7 Hopeful Facts About Stroke)

Stand Up to Stroke

Strike Back At Stroke

Stroke—Why Do They Behave That Way

Take Care of Your Heart

Ten Commandments for the Patient with High Blood Pressure—Wallet Card

Thank You for Not Smoking—Posters

Tin Woodman 'Take Care of Your Heart' Coloring Book

Up and Around, A Booklet to Aid the Stroke Patient In Activities of Daily Living

Usted y Su Corazon (You and Your Heart)

Varicose Veins

Wallet Card—Emergency Action—Nitroglycerin

Way to A Man's Heart, A Fat-Controlled, Low-Cholesterol Meal Plan to Reduce the Risk of Heart Attack

A LIST OF MATERIALS FOR THE PUBLIC (Cont.)

Weight Control Guidance in Smoking Cessation	What Goes Up Must Come Down—Poster
What Everyone Should Know About Smoking and Heart Disease	You, Your Child and Rheumatic Fever
	Your Heart And How It Works—Chart
What Every Woman Should Know About High Blood Pressure	Your Heart And How It works—Diagram

INDEX